About the authors

Carol Leverkus BSc, SRD started her career with *Slimming magazine* and from 1977 worked in South Bedfordshire Health Authority developing the Community Dietetic Service. She also works part-time as a freelance nutrition advisor. She served on the Community Nutrition Group Committee from 1980–1984.

Isobel Cole-Hamilton BSc, SRD, works as Project Officer with the London Food Commission. She spent 7 years as a Community Dietitian in Lambeth. During that time she was on the BDA Council and she also chaired the Community Nutrition Group. She is co-author of the *Nutrition Guidelines* produced by the ILEA.

Karen Gunner MSc, SRD worked as a hospital dietitian, then as a Nutrition Consultant in Montreal, Canada. In this country she has worked as a dietitian, and in Health Education in Richmond and Kingston, before joining Burson Marsteller, a public relations consultancy in London.

Jennifer Starr BSc, SRD is currently the District Dietitian for the Eastbourne Health Authority. She is an active member of the British Dietetic Association and joined the Community Nutrition Group 7 years ago.

Dr Andrew Stanway MB, MRCP practised medicine on the Professorial Medical Unit at King's Hospital in London before leaving to edit medical journals for doctors for five years. He has written seventeen book .... with his wife, Dr Penny Stanway, the bestsell .... *is Best*; and *Taking the Rough with* .... Surrey.

Also available from Century

THE
GREAT BRITISH DIET

*Dietitians and their families test a recipe
for healthy eating*

Carol Leverkus
Isobel Cole-Hamilton
Karen Gunner
Jennifer Starr
with
Dr Andrew Stanway MB, MRCP

CENTURY PUBLISHING
LONDON

Nothing in this book should be taken to be official policy of the
British Dietetic Association – it is the work and opinion of the
authors unless otherwise stated.

First published in Great Britain in 1985
by Century Hutchinson Ltd,
Brookmount House,
62–65 Chandos Place, London WC2N 4NW

ISBN 0 7126 1033 2

Photoset by Rowland Phototypesetting Ltd
Bury St Edmunds, Suffolk
Printed in Great Britain in 1985 by
Hunt Barnard Printing Ltd, Aylesbury, Bucks

Acknowledgements

We are extremely grateful to all the participants in this study and to Professor Michael Crawford, Wendy Doyle and Patrick Drury for their valuable consultations and time given on all aspects of the research, particularly their extensive computer analyses. Thanks are extended to the dietitians who coded the food records and to the Flora Project for Heart Disease Prevention for their support in sponsoring the vital computer and analytical work.

The advice and support of Greta Walton, Chairman of the BDA until May 1985 and Alison Black, of the Dunn Nutrition unit, Cambridge, has been greatly appreciated as has the help with the lifestyle questionnaires and interviews from: R. Watson, Queen Elizabeth College London and Julia Parsons, Ann Heughan, Joan Scriven and Hazel Coubrough (dietitians).

Without the understanding, advice and support of Alan Starr, Peter Leverkus and David Gunner this large research project and the book would have been impossible.

We thank you all.

Contents

Introduction

Food and eating are complex and emotive issues, involving, as they do, so much more than simply nourishing ourselves. Food has important social, ritual and even sexual connotations – indeed getting people to talk about the intricacies of their eating habits is much like asking them to share details of their sex lives. This is hardly surprising because eating and sex are man's two most powerful drives. The first ensures the survival of the individual and the second that of the species.

Because there are so many social overtones to food and eating, and probably always have been throughout history, there are as many views about eating as there are people who eat. Most people consider themselves to be experts on eating and all of us have our pet theories about which foods are good for us and how they affect us.

Until about 150 years ago the problem for most ordinary people was getting enough good quality food to fill their stomachs and nourish them adequately. The body needs a minimum supply of proteins, fats, carbohydrates, vitamins and minerals to work properly and to repair itself both during natural wear and tear and after illness. If a person becomes too low in any one of the vital nutrients he will suffer from a deficiency disease, scurvy in the case of Vitamin C, for example. Such obvious deficiency states have been recognised for 200 years but in more recent times more subtle deficiencies have been found and doubtless many more are yet to be discovered. The current vogue is for minerals and other trace nutrients. Research over many decades in animals has found that they are deficient in certain trace elements. Just how such deficiencies apply to humans is not yet known but it is a subject of increasing interest in medical and scientific articles. This could just be another dietary fashion or it could be the start of new and exciting insights into all kinds of ailments and diseases.

Some foods are rich in many nutrients and others in only a few very specific ones and it was a knowledge and understanding of this that led to the concept of a 'balanced diet'.

This concept was developed to prevent deficiency diseases and was most vigorously promoted during and after World War II. The idea behind such a diet was to make sure that most people *didn't go short* of what were then recognised to be essential nutrients. Such an emphasis was understandable – indeed it has occurred more recently with the rediscovery of dietary fibre in the 1970s. Once the scientific fraternity finds that a particular foodstuff is essential for health, and indeed life, they understandably promote it and the food industry produces it. So it was with the discovery of vitamins and minerals in the early part of this century. Suddenly it became 'vital' to choose foods and balance them to provide what was thought to be a balanced diet for the average man-in-the-street.

Such thinking also led to what we now know to be an over-emphasis on nutrients. Every schoolchild knows that we need proteins, fats, carbohydrates, minerals and vitamins, and the up-to-date ones will add dietary fibre to the list. But nutrition education at every level, even that of professionals, has tended to stress the division of foods into these pigeon holes, often very unhelpfully. For example, 'protein foods' are said to be good for growth and repair; 'energy foods' for work; and 'protective foods' (vitamins and minerals) to keep us healthy over all. A food such as sugar, which is pure energy, has been seen as acceptable because it could be 'balanced' by other more nutritious foods.

Such groupings are now seen as somewhat misleading because no single food group does one thing in the body. The truth is that many foods provide not only energy but other valuable substances. Such a classification also arbitrarily misplaces foods in categories into which they don't fit in the light of today's knowledge. For years cheese has been regarded as good, wholesome protein, whereas in reality it is a high-fat food and we all already consume far too much fat.

So the old concept of a balanced diet is now outdated. According to most doctors, few, except the very poor and the very frail elderly, suffer from nutritional deficiency diseases in the UK. The truth may in fact be rather different, as we shall see. What is certain though is that we tend to eat too much of the wrong things.

The Fashion for Slimness and Health

Food, like so many other things in societies around the world, is subject to fashion. Today in the West, slimness is all the rage, partly from a health viewpoint and partly for aesthetic reasons. 'Diets' abound and a book such as Audrey Eyton's *F-Plan Diet* has been bought and read avidly by millions – mainly women who are keen to be in fashion and slim.

Unfortunately, almost all diet books are bound to fail, except in publishing terms, because people are being asked to give up things they like and we have already mentioned how primitive a business eating really is. People want to eat what they like and like what they eat and anything that takes them away from this principle will make them feel virtuous (and slim) but only for a while. Alas, for many people the old conditioning, social pressures, unsuitability of many processed foods and so on all militate against them and soon they find they are back to eating as they used to. Some people – hundreds and thousands of them – run their lives like this year in and year out clinging on to the latest slimming fashion which is a supposedly healthy way to eat.

Over the last decade in the UK, and perhaps twice that long in the USA, there has been an increasing awareness of the link between general health and what we eat. Numerous studies have shown the dangers of overweight; that cancers can be caused by diet; that we eat too little dietary fibre; and that we eat too much sugar, fat and so on. You would need a very substantial warehouse to contain all the scientific and medical research about diet and health that has appeared over the last 20 years alone.

Yet for all this publicity most of us eat very unhealthily. A number of surveys conducted in the USA and in the UK have found that the 'balanced diet' is largely a myth. In 1980 the Bateman Organisation conducted an in-depth survey in the UK into people's eating habits and found that only 15 per cent were eating a diet that contained even the minimum suggestions laid down by the DHSS. In the USA two researchers looked at 800 patients attending a dental hospital. Half were deficient in Vitamin C and 6 per cent had no Vitamin C in their blood at all. Another study of 120 randomly selected patients in a New Jersey medical centre found that 88 per cent had a significant deficiency of at least one vitamin and that 63 per cent were deficient in two or more vitamins.

Just why our so-called 'balanced diet' is in fact so unbalanced is a complex story, the answers to which will become apparent in the course of this book.

The British Dietetic Association (BDA) Study

The British Dietetic Association, the professional body representing the country's dietitians, could see what was happening to British nutrition. What people were actually eating was already well known from the various surveys and other work carried out by the National Food Survey and other nutrition research bodies. However, the BDA also wanted to see what could be achieved by altering people's whole eating patterns to something more healthy. They were not looking for another 'diet' in the accepted sense of the word but for ways of encouraging people to eat more healthily on a permanent basis.

This book is the result of a unique study carried out in 1984 among dietitians and their families in the UK. The study is a milestone in nutritional and dietary thinking because for the first time on any large scale, real-life families were involved in a highly detailed analysis of their normal eating and nutrition, both before and after trying to eat according to a new set of goals for healthier eating.

These goals were those set by the National Advisory Committee on Nutrition Education (NACNE) which was instituted in 1979 by the British Nutrition Foundation and the Health Education Council.

The BDA study was originally intended to provide professional information and to draw up simple guidelines to help the public achieve healthy eating goals. So valuable were its findings and the experiences of the participants, however, that we decided to share them with the general public.

CHAPTER ONE

The Story Behind the NACNE Report

For years various governments had realised that the public and the health and nutrition professions were thoroughly confused about dietary advice. Almost every year, it seemed, another learned paper or book set up a new hypothesis or demolished an old one and the public were at a loss to know how to eat. Industry, the government, the professions and the media all appeared to contradict one another and the man-in-the-street was caught between them all. The result all too often was simply 'A plague on all your houses – I'll eat what I like.'

As a result of all this confusion, and in an effort to get some sense out of it all a government working party was set up in 1973 which included members from the Department of Health & Social Security (DHSS): the Health Education Council (HEC) which is funded by government; and the British Nutrition Foundation (BNF) which is funded by the food industry. The main recommendation of this working party was that there was an urgent need for simple and accurate information on nutrition.

In parallel with the setting up of the working party in the UK, Senator George McGovern in the USA was already working towards his report *Dietary Goals for the United States* which was issued in 1977. This was a forward-looking document that laid out the bald facts: that most Americans were eating too much fat, sugar and salt, and that this was linked to increased death rates from various western diseases. Since then 13 countries have followed suit and produced their own nutritional guidelines.

The National Advisory Committee on Nutrition Education

(NACNE) was set up in Britain in 1979 as a direct result of the working party mentioned above. Professor J. N. Morris, a highly experienced doctor involved in public health, was appointed chairman. Various other interested parties also had their say on NACNE. There were representatives of the DHSS, the Ministry of Agriculture (MAFF), spokesmen from the food industry, and of course people from the Health Education Council. In the early days there was quite a lot of conflict because these rather different groups had such different viewpoints. It would be quite wrong to suggest that this was just the food industry versus the rest (as has been suggested) – there were, and still are, mainstream dietary experts who didn't find it easy to agree.

It became apparent that a simple authoritative statement was necessary to clear things up so the vice chairman of NACNE, Dr (now Professor) Philip James, was asked to draw one up. It was agreed that 'clear and simple messages were necessary, and unambiguous advice that could be put into practice by the public.'

Dr James, an eminent nutritionist, now head of the Rowatt Research Institute in Scotland, gathered around him a group of experts to help him. These people then sorted through the main publications in the field and came down on eight expert, national and international committee reports, which they used as the basis for their own Report. These eight documents were:

1 *Eating for Health*, DHSS, 1978, 1979: HMSO
2 *Diet and coronary heart disease*, the DHSS Report on Health and Social Subjects No. 7, 1974: HMSO
3 *Prevention of Coronary Artery Disease*, Joint Report of the Royal College of Physicians and the British Cardiac Society, 1976
4 *Medical Aspects of Dietary Fibre*, Report of the Royal College of Physicians, 1981: Pitman
5 *Recommended daily amounts of food energy and nutrients for groups of people in the United Kingdom*, DHSS Report on Health and Social Subjects No. 15, 1979: HMSO
6 *Avoiding Heart Attacks*, The DHSS Report, 1981: HMSO

7 *Prevention of Coronary Heart Disease*, WHO Report, 1982: WHO

8 *Obesity*, Report of the Royal College of Physicians, 1983

In April 1981 Dr James submitted his final draft of the document requested by NACNE but there were two problems. The first was that, given the brief they had to work to, it was no longer acceptable to go along with old concepts about diet information. The 'new' ideas implied in this were that first, we are all at risk from eating badly – it's not just a problem for the elderly, the pregnant or the immigrant population – as had been previously portrayed by doctors and nutritionists. Second, it became clear that general, wishy-washy advice about eating 'some of this' and 'less of that' were now useless and simply hadn't worked. It was very obvious that people needed real goals to aim for.

All of this is difficult enough to achieve, but when there are parties on a committee with very different views, achieving a consensus that they can all go along with is difficult, to put it mildly. These disagreements continued over much of 1982 and 1983 during which time there were several revisions of the Report. Dr James and his colleagues tried to accommodate all the points of view expressed by the committee and many other expert views were incorporated into the document. But progress was very slow. During this time certain doctors and health educators became aware of the impact of the McGovern Report in the USA and were aware of the long process the Americans went through before having their report recognised and implemented. However, after a very few years it was clear that changes in lifestyle including eating habits were producing positive results in the nation's health and that the heart disease death rate was falling steadily.

In the UK, where nutrition has always been something of a Cinderella in the medical world, people were continuing to suffer unnecessarily from diseases on which other countries were making an impact, and a few knowledgeable health professionals found this hard to accept. One went so far as to say that the delays in the publication of NACNE amounted to 'the biggest scandal in British public health since the Victorian days when officials refused to accept or act on the fact that cholera and typhoid are water-borne diseases.'

In April 1983 Dr James submitted his fourth draft of the NACNE Report. This was not published. As a result, the media, and in particular the *Sunday Times* newspaper took a special interest in the subject.

The next milestone, and probably the most vital in this story, came in the form of a series of articles on nutrition in the learned medical journal – *The Lancet*. It started a series of features entitled 'Nutrition: the changing scene'. For the first time a major medical journal accepted the fact that most of our Western diseases are diet-related and by implication dragged the medical profession screaming into the dietary debates of the 1980s. At last doctors were forced to admit that diet played a crucial role in the causation of disease. This seems common-sense to most members of the public who understandably express amazement that doctors did not, until very recently, believe it to be so. Eventually, *The Lancet* published the NACNE Report as four long extracts and began a new era of nutrition education. The general feeling among doctors, scientists and the press was that the suggestions in the Report were so important and far-reaching for society as a whole that they should be publicised at once.

The NACNE Report finally saw the light of day in September 1983 when it was published by the Health Education Council.

What did NACNE Recommend?

First of all it is important to point out exactly what the NACNE Report was and what it wasn't. It was a discussion document aimed at health and nutrition professionals to give them guidelines on which to structure nutrition education. It was *not* meant as a new sort of 'diet' to be taken up *en masse* by the public.

The NACNE Report acknowledged that any change in eating patterns would have to be achieved slowly and gently. As a result they divided their recommendations into short- and long-term goals. The long-term goals were to be implemented during the 1980s and 1990s; the short-term ones to be achieved within five years.

The Long-term Goals

- The recommendations are for the population as a whole and *not* for individuals. Groups such as immigrants, children, the elderly and pregnant women may need additional advice. We are all at risk from the typical western diet.
- On balance, **overweight** people should not be eating less but exercising more. They should also change their eating patterns.
- **Smoking** is more dangerous than overweight but ex-smokers should also exercise more and change their eating patterns.
- **Fat** consumption should be cut by one quarter, to 30 per cent of total energy intake from the present level of 38 per cent.
- **Saturated fat** should be cut by nearly one half to 10 per cent of total energy intake from the current level of 18 per cent.
- There is no recommendation to increase the amount of **polyunsaturated fat** eaten. The proportions of polyunsaturates to saturates will rise as the amount of saturates falls.
- There is no change recommended in **cholesterol** intake.
- **Sugar** consumption should be cut by nearly one half – from 38kg to 20kg per person per year (this does not include other added sugars such as glucose and glucose syrups). Consumption of **sugar in snacks** should be no more than half of total sugar intake – this means 10kg per person per year.
- **Fibre** consumption for adults should be increased by one half, to 30g a day from the current level of about 20g. Fibre should be eaten as wholefoods, cereals and vegetables and fruit.
- **Salt** consumption should be cut by 3g a day from the current level of 8–12g. Most people's intake is probably nearer the higher figure.
- **Alcohol** consumption should be cut by one third to 4 per

cent of total energy intake from the present level of 6 per cent.

● There is no recommendation about the amount of **protein** eaten. Overall, animal protein should be eaten less and plant protein more.

● There is no recommendation to alter the current level of **vitamins and minerals** from those laid down as recommended daily allowances (RDAs) by the DHSS.

● There is a definite need for clear, informative **labelling of foods** so that people can see at a glance details of energy, sugars, salt, fibre and the different types of fats.

The Short-term Goals

Realising that such changes could not be achieved quickly yet also understanding the need to do *something* sooner rather than later, NACNE drew up a list of goals or targets that could be implemented at once by anyone who really wanted to do so. These short-term goals achieve about one third of the total long-term goals.

● **Fat** Cut consumption by 10 per cent overall. Saturated fats should be cut by 15 per cent and polyunsaturated fat consumption increased by a quarter to 5 per cent of total energy intake.

● **Sugar** Cut down by 10 per cent. Slowly reduce and eventually stop adding sugar to drinks. Cut right down on sugary snacks.

● **Energy** Take more exercise.

● **Fibre** Increase by one quarter. This is easy to do simply by replacing white bread with wholemeal and having a whole-of-the-grain breakfast cereal every day.

● **Salt** Cut down by 10 per cent – in other words, by 1g a day. Slowly wean yourself off salt at the table.

● **Alcohol** Cut down by 16 per cent.

All of these short-term changes can be achieved easily by modifying what you eat. They don't necessarily involve any revolutions in eating patterns and habits, don't require Acts of Parliament or changes within the food industry and are easily achieved by the average person who wants to improve his or her health.

In summary then the NACNE Report could be said to have summarised all the best available nutritional evidence and come up with the following recommendations:

- Eat more whole, fresh food, preferably of vegetable origin.
- Eat more bread (preferably wholemeal), potatoes, cereals, vegetables and fruit.
- Eat fish, lean red meat and poultry and fewer dairy products.
- Eat less processed food generally.

Why Bother About NACNE? Isn't it Just Another Fad?

Readers could be forgiven for thinking that the NACNE Report was just another here-today-gone-tomorrow medical fashion but they would be wrong and for several reasons.

NACNE is not, of course, the last word on nutrition but neither is it a 'fashionable' document. It draws together all the best evidence from international studies and interprets it cautiously and sensibly. It represents the best consensus of opinion that there is. But this doesn't make it the Gospel truth. First, there are several errors and omissions. Sugar consumption, for example, only reflected sucrose intake and not the consumption of other sugars added to food and drink. Sucrose is the brown or white sugar we normally use and is added commercially to many foods. Second, new research findings are hitting the medical headlines every month and these will naturally make the experts think again. Third, because NACNE was designed to apply to whole population groups on average, as opposed to individuals, it can't be directly applied to any one person. What *can* be generally said is that almost all of us need to eat less sugar, saturated fat and salt and more fibre. Last, whatever changes individuals make to their own ways of eating the real decisions lie in the hands of governments and the food industry, both of whom have so much control over the foods we actually have to choose from.

Since NACNE the Government Report *Diet and Cardiovascular Disease* has been produced by the Committee on Medical Aspects of Food Policy (COMA). This 1984 report made recommendations similar to NACNE, particularly on dietary fats, but was, unlike NACNE, restricting itself to heart disease.

There is now so much evidence that food is linked to the incidence of various diseases that even the most head-in-the-sand individual can no longer overlook NACNE-type advice completely. The following summarises what is known of the link between foods and illnesses.

Disease	Associated with excess	Associated with too little
Obesity	Fat, sugar, calorie intake	Fibre
Tooth decay	Sugar	Fibre
Digestive system:		
constipation		Fibre
diverticular disease		Fibre
cancer of the colon	Fat	Fibre
gall bladder disease	Calorie intake, fat	Fibre
Heart and blood vessels:		
heart disease	Fat, calorie intake	
high blood pressure	Calorie intake, salt	
stroke	Calorie intake, salt	
Breast cancer	Fat	
Stomach cancer	Salt	
Diabetes, maturity onset	Calorie intake	

What surprises many people is that given that the link between the food we eat and western killer diseases is so well-documented, they have not heard about all this before now. The reality is that research over the last ten to fifteen years looking at disease patterns around the world has found that most western diseases appear to be closely linked to eating habits. As people move from rural societies with traditional diets to the West, or as they adopt western eating habits, they begin to experience our western diseases. Slowly the pieces of the jigsaw fitted together to produce links between disease and eating which were, until recently, simply elegant theories suggested by a few forward-thinking individuals. There is now no doubt that healthy eating is one of the most important weapons we have against most western diseases. In other words the uncontrolled 'trials' that have been done as populations around the world adopt our western eating habits have proved without doubt that the way we eat produces illnesses. By extending this argument, returning to a more traditional way of eating reduces the burden of disease in a society.

Many people have criticised the food industry for producing unwholesome food. But is this fair? The industry claim to produce what we, the public are prepared to buy and will only continue to produce what people will buy. Only ten years ago millers and bakers were maintaining that wholemeal bread couldn't be made as widely available as white bread for a host of (to them) very convincing reasons. A trip around any supermarket today proves how silly this stance was yet similar postures are being taken by certain sectors of the food industry today about other unfamiliar foods. The reality is that eating will never be the same again in this country as a result of the NACNE Report and forward-thinking food companies know this only too well. Indeed, in today's nutritional climate there's considerable mileage to be made in public relations terms by companies who lead the way in producing healthier foods. To be fair to them the problem the industry has often had is knowing which way to jump. Changes in production lines involve vast expenditures, as do the marketing and advertising of new products. With medical advice changing so rapidly it has often been near impossible for the industry to know exactly what to make – always bearing in mind that their first responsibility is to their shareholders.

Until healthy food becomes an integral part of government policy progress is bound to be patchy. Individuals can only do so much, which puts the onus on the food industry and the Government to make serious, far-reaching changes. This involves the catering, farming, food distribution, political, manufacturing, health and educational sectors of society which together employ millions of people. Changes are bound to affect all of them as employees as well just as members of the public.

Major changes in any area of life take a generation or two to come about but at least with food we can all make our own individual starts both personally in our own homes and by putting pressure on the food industry and the Government by encouraging them to produce what we want to eat. Neither farmers nor the food industry want to resist change as a matter of principle. As a leader of an American farmers' union put it, 'My members want protection from heart attacks every bit as much as everyone else.'

CHAPTER TWO

The Background to the BDA Study

The study took its final form in the spring of 1984 and had its origins at a meeting of the Committee of the Community Nutrition Group of the British Dietetic Association in the winter of 1981. This was more than two years before the publication of NACNE.

But before we go any further it will probably be helpful if we outline briefly a little about The British Dietetic Association and see who dietitians are and what they do.

What is the British Dietetic Association?

The BDA was formed in 1936. It is the professional association for qualified dietitians in the UK and an independent trade union.

The BDA aims to: advance the science and practice of dietetics and associated subjects by promoting the training and education of dietitians; spread the knowledge and further understanding of dietetics; facilitate the exchange of information and views among members of the Association and other professional and lay people; co-operate with similar professional bodies in the UK, EEC countries and elsewhere in the world.

To fulfil these aims the BDA has a governing Council of elected members with various supporting Committees and its own scientific journal *Human Nutrition: Applied Nutrition*. On a less formal note it provides a forum for the exchange of news and views through a newsletter which is sent to members each month. The BDA currently has over 1800 members.

Who are Dietitians?

Contrary to popular opinion, dietitians spend only a small part of their time advising people how to lose weight. Their work interests range from hospitals to industry, public relations, research and the local community. Such a wide spectrum demands specialist training over a period of years. All qualified dietitians hold a degree or diploma, recognised for State Registration by the Council for Professions Supplementary to Medicine. Since 1981, dietetics has become an all-degree profession and entry qualifications are a minimum of two A-levels, including chemistry and another science. All diplomas are now postgraduate ones.

Over the past decade, dietetics has become a more authoritative, vocal and self-confident profession. Dietitians are predominantly women (a ratio of 60 women to each man) with the majority employed in the National Health Service. Traditionally, dietitians worked in hospitals and were concerned only with therapeutic diets. This is still the largest part of the profession's work, but increasingly, Health Service-employed dietitians are also active within the general community. Some BDA members are employed in influential positions outside the Health Service and as freelance dietitians.

What Does a Therapeutic Dietitian do?

The modification of a patient's diet may often be an integral part of his or her medical treatment, such as for diabetes or heart disease. It is the dietitian's role to provide this specialist service at the request of physicians, surgeons or general practitioners. The dietitian is then subsequently responsible for teaching patients about their diet and for helping them to make it as varied and palatable as possible. They can then enjoy their food and at the same time fit in with the eating patterns of their families and friends as much as possible. Following a diet for a few weeks, especially one that is recommended for a 'medical' condition, can seriously try the patience of most people; to follow one for life needs a lot of support and it is this support that dietitians are trained to give.

Therapeutic dietitians are increasingly making their presence felt around the hospital. They are now also helping staff and patients to recognise the importance of food in the prevention of disease. When it comes to the treatment of special conditions dietitians have an assured future.

Dietitians and Dietary Change

Why has the dietetic profession not been as successful at promoting dietary change as one might expect?

First, when it comes to food and public health, dietitians are not well established at a national level, although this situation is slowly changing. Locally, many dietitians are involved in advising both Health and Education Authorities and companies on nutrition policies. Better representation nationally is what is really required to bring about the fundamental changes that will improve all of our diets. Examples include influencing food laws, national policies or the food prepared in government institutions (the Government is the largest cook in Britain, when you consider all the institutions it controls).

Second, dietitians are largely dependent on the enthusiasm of other people to help carry out their ideas.

As we saw earlier, most dietitians are female. Indeed, the profession is largely made up of young women and the career structure which has developed has not necessarily encouraged dietitians to reach senior positions of authority. Whatever the causes of this state of affairs, this in addition presents dietitians with a difficult task when trying to influence food policies, whether at local or national level. This has undoubtedly been a negative factor in changing the nation's eating habits.

Whilst the work of the BDA and its individual members is increasingly bringing dietetics to people's attention, there is still more work to be done. For example, even within the NHS the spread of dietetic influence is limited – nutrition has yet to become a mandatory part of the syllabus in medical schools and most doctors still see food, and thus dietitians, as less than vital in the battle to prevent disease and ill health.

Dietitians' training is becoming increasingly scientific which is helping their image in the eyes of the medical profession – particularly those working in hospitals. But this scientific basis is not in itself helping to overcome the problem of 'spreading the word about healthy eating'. Eight universities, colleges and polytechnics in the United Kingdom offer degree or postgraduate courses in nutrition and dietetics. These courses cover such scientific subjects as food science, medicine, physiology, biochemistry, microbiology and nutrition. Not all courses, however, adequately prepare dietitians on the psycho-social aspects of nutrition and health. As food is such an important· part of our everyday lives, a grasp of these aspects is essential when advising dietary change. Recognising this problem, the BDA is currently investigating ways of implementing postgraduate training for community dietitians. Similarly, dietitians following a career outside the NHS such as in industry or the media, could benefit from better preparation for their work.

Interest in Healthy Eating Within the NHS

Advice about healthy eating did not start with NACNE. Prior to the publication of the NACNE Report some Health Authorities had begun to draw up and even adopt nutrition policies aimed at promoting the health of people of all ages within their boundaries. This action is now being increasingly taken by more authorities.

When this is done in a hospital setting it has to involve a wide range of personnel and disciplines, including caterers, nursing staff, dietitians, housekeepers, medical staff, voluntary services and supplies service staff. The dietitian is thus one amongst many who will have a part to play in the everyday implementation of such a policy. It will be the responsibility of a nurse to order a patient's meals and it is largely the role of the caterer to produce appetising menus and tasty meals.

This does not mean that dietitians are powerless but that they tend to have an overall advisory role. This is where their political skills come to the fore. For example, through nutrition policies they are obtaining the support of the Health Authorities' Management Teams – giving more clout to their advisory role. As a more specific example, dietitians may be instrumental in ensuring that the health promotion aspects of catering are included in the job description of a new caterer.

Healthy Eating Programmes Outside the NHS

Many Health Authorities now see it as their wider brief to try to encourage other services such as Education and Social Services to adopt sound nutrition practices and examples of this can be seen around the country.

The initiative to provide a choice of healthy food in the workplace is also being taken up by groups of workers in many different companies.

Occupational health staff, catering and personnel staff and many enthusiastic individuals are increasingly turning to dietitians and other health workers for advice and suggestions, so leading to changes in the types of food available, particularly for workers.

Above all, the general public has become increasingly concerned with the issues of diet and health. Books and magazines on the subject abound.

The impetus for change is coming from a wide range of people; but change will need more than the efforts of dietitians, members of the nursing and medical professions and interested individuals. It will also require a change on the part of the food industry and government, where to date little movement has been seen.

As happens in almost any sphere of life today, things have become so complex that specialisation is essential. Dietetics is no exception. The therapeutic side has developed its own specialities and the BDA now has several groups with specific areas of interest.

Of the 670 members in these specialist groups 190 are particularly concerned with community nutrition, and it is dietitians from this group who were responsible for this study.

The Community Nutrition Group (CNG)

The CNG of the BDA is made up of qualified, state-registered dietitians working in various aspects of nutrition education. It was formed to give an opportunity to exchange views and give support to its members, who were often working 'in professional isolation'. This isolation was especially real (compared with, say, dietitians working in hospitals and other institutions) because it is very rare for a Health Authority to employ more than one community dietitian.

What do Community Dietitians do?

The majority of CNG members are employed as Community Dietitians in the NHS. A handful work as Health Education Officers, again within the NHS. Small numbers work as community dietitians/nutritionists for Social Services, for food companies, as nutrition and dietetic lecturers, or in research. A few also work for various organisations and authorities, including one for the DHSS. More than a dozen are employed in freelance work, such as writing books, or as consultants to catering firms and food companies, or in writing for the media.

Since 1974 Health Authorities have been gradually employing more dietitians to work in the Community Health Service. This has been a positive step towards improving this country's diet and health. This kind of work in the preventive area involves promoting knowledge about the dietary inadvisability of saturated fats and refined foods and the sort of problems that await us on the supermarket shelves. The community dietitian's work is to help persuade the general public that good health depends on eating more fibre from cereals, vegetables and fruit, together with eating more fish, beans and lean meat rather than the fatty foods. The work has a strong public relations slant to it and frequently involves writing leaflets for local use. They liaise with health visitors and other community nurses, GPs, social workers, ethnic minority leaders and other local groups and organisations. It is most likely to be the community dietitian who will turn up to give an illustrated talk to a women's or a pre-retirement group. Typically they would help with the general or special diet menus at a residential house.

A community dietitian's work encompasses a wide range of responsibilities requiring good communication skills. In other words, she or he needs to make academic-sounding advice actually work in schools, hospitals, colleges and in individuals' homes.

The Community Nutrition Group's members have, since its foundation in 1972, set themselves the task of investigating controversial areas of nutrition and dietetics for the use of all BDA members, other professionals, and indeed members of the public.

It was in this context that the CNG took responsibility for translating the NACNE goals into foods which we could all eat.

How the Study was Born

December 1981
Committee members of the CNG of the BDA agreed that the meeting to be held in April 1983 should try to gain a consensus of opinion from the members attending the meeting on whether dietary goals for the population should or should not be pursued and if so, what the membership thought these goals should be. It was anticipated that some people from outside the BDA would attend, as it was agreed that other interested parties could contribute a lot to such a discussion. As a result, teachers and home economists, among others, were encouraged to attend.

December 1981–April 1983
Arrangements were made for the meeting and a set of topics were presented on the day to be discussed with a view to developing dietary goals from them. The topics discussed are listed below with the two questions to be discussed.

1 Should there be dietary goals for:
   infant feeding practices

energy balance
dietary fibre intake
fat consumption
sugar consumption
salt consumption
animal and vegetable protein consumption
alcohol consumption
intake of food additives
individual nutrients
relative proportions of protein, fat and carbohydrate in the diet?

2 Could the experts agree on whether there should be dietary goals?

April 1983

Northwick Park Hospital hosted a meeting of CNG members and certain key people involved in nutrition education in London. For all of those involved this proved to be very exciting – at the end of the day we had all agreed to the way forward. To achieve this all those attending were allocated to one of eleven working groups to consider a particular topic in depth and then to report back to the meeting for discussion.

The encouraging outcome was the high level of agreement reached amongst those attending. This led to a Press statement being issued to try to publicise the fact that professionals could agree about nutrition!

The meeting also specified that the general recommendations reached would need further investigation for all groups within the population who might be at a special nutritional risk, for example, children, pregnant women, the elderly and ethnic minority groups.

So before the publication of NACNE we had shown the level of agreement amongst professionals when looking at dietary changes over a ten- to fifteen-year period. We had highlighted the need for goals to work towards.

At the end of the day ten people arranged to meet to follow these issues up. So the BDA had agreed that dietary goals were a good idea. But could they put them into practice?

May–October 1983

Now reduced to ten – and all enthusiastic to continue with examining the practicality of dietary goals for the population as a whole – where were the BDA to go next? They now had a set of dietary goals to aim for, but how could they apply them to the general public? How could they find out about the difficulties individuals might well experience in changing their eating habits and their choice of foods to meet such goals? Would it be possible to suggest that each individual ate a particular number of slices of bread? Could we ever answer people's questions about how much of a certain food to eat?

It was decided that each of the ten members of the group should seek the co-operation of three individuals, so that it would be possible to study the eating patterns and food intakes of thirty people. Each person agreeing to participate was asked to keep an accurate record of their food intake for a week. This involved writing down details of all the food and drink that passed their lips during one week by either recording a weight, if given on a packet or tin, or giving a description of the food in terms of portion size. The more accurate the description, the more accurate the analysis could be.

For example, a breakfast listed as:

cereals and milk
toast, butter,
marmalade and coffee

would be much more helpful if recorded in the following way:

1oz Weetabix
1 cup silver top milk
2 large slices medium cut, white loaf
butter spread thickly
2 teaspoons thick-cut marmalade
coffee with a dash of silver top milk
2 teaspoons sugar.

The dietitian could then:

quantify the food records

arrange for the food diaries to be analysed, and
draw up guidelines for each individual based on the analysis
of their food records.

The dietitians hoped that each of the thirty people would try to
act on this advice, to eat in a way which was consistent with the
guidelines prepared for them to keep a record of a second
week's food intake to see how they managed.

As a result of discussions with the people participating, the
research group hoped to gain some idea of the changes people
had found in the second week. For example:

Did they enjoy their food in this week?
Had they had to alter where they ate?
Was there any change in their food bill?

As is often the case, none of this proved to be quite so easy in
practice. This was partly because:

• Incomplete food records made analysis of the food intakes inaccurate.
• Even where good records had been well recorded it
proved difficult for the dietitians organising the project to
obtain the computer facilities necessary for analysing the
data.
• The individual records were analysed with different data
so it was difficult to compare like with like.
• Very few participants were able to complete the second
week of the project and in some cases contact was lost with
the participants.

This initial project emphasised the need for a far more methodical and precise approach using many more participants and
proved that if any headway was to be made at all a better-
planned, more scientific study was needed. A good deal more
thought also needed to be given to investigating factors which
affect food choice. As with many other areas related to the
adoption of a healthy lifestyle we may *know* what is better for
us but we do not always follow the advice.

What are the Pressures Affecting Food Choice?

Social, economic and psychological factors usually have more to do with a person's food choice and the amount of food eaten than does its nutritional value. Religious and cultural traditions, social conventions, peer group pressures, household influences, individual preferences and priorities, habits, lifestyles and nutritional knowledge are all seen as influencing our choice of diet. Additionally, the cost and availability of certain foods are affected by region, Government policies and subsidies, agricultural practice, the policy of manufacturing industries, and by distribution systems.

Here are some of the specific problems encountered and the ways in which the group of dietitians involved thought they could be overcome.

Increased cost of some foods e.g. leaner cuts of meat, low-fat cheeses	Changes in pricing policies by Government and the food industry
Changes in taste unpopular e.g. less salt and sugar	Gradual change, use of alternative flavourings
Misconceptions about food e.g. 'should eat meat every day' 'need sugar for energy' 'bread and cereals are fattening'	Education and advertising about food and health
Unfamiliar tastes are often disliked and social conventions may make it difficult to change	Give a variety of tastes from an early age and try to change gradually through education e.g. introduce in institutions
Availability of cheap, convenient meals for preparation at home and for purchase outside	Development by the food industry
Availability of suitable snack foods	Development by the food industry

Availability of suitable foods in the works canteen, local cafés and restaurants	Changes in the catering industry. Government establishments could take a lead as the Government is the largest cook
Lack of practical nutrition education in catering colleges	Move to encourage preparation of healthy meal choices in the kitchen as well as in the classroom

In September 1983, as we saw earlier, the NACNE report was published and the issues raised by this document, together with the work which had been going on by members of the BDA, reinforced dietitians' beliefs that the practicality of such measures needed to be tested and that dietitians were the group of professionals with the expertise to do this. The dietitians involved in this study thus took their findings and ideas back to other BDA members before proceeding any further.

October 1983

The CNG meeting agreed to ask the BDA to fund a research project to investigate the practicality of eating to the NACNE goals. A protocol outlining the study was to be prepared and it was agreed that the participants this time should be dietitians and adult members of their households before any further attempts were made to look at the eating habits of the general public. This was because dietitians would not need to be taught how to try and change their diet to achieve the goals. One of the aims of the study was to be able to come up with guidelines on which to base teaching materials for the public.

The difficulties we had encountered in our initial attempt had helped to identify the following points:

1 A detailed, methodical approach was needed.
2 Computer facilities were needed for accurate dietary analyses.
3 Dietitians should be used in the study as they have the knowledge needed to make the necessary changes in their

eating habits and lifestyles even to stand a chance of attaining the NACNE goals.

4 The long-term NACNE goals should be the target set.

As the computer facilities were a stumbling block it was an enormous help when the Flora Project for Heart Disease Prevention provided the BDA with the computer time for this expensive analytical work.

All that remained now was to see how good dietitians would be at eating their own words!

January 1984

Four members (the dietitian authors of this book) continued to meet and prepare the research project which was presented to, and accepted by, the BDA in spring 1984. Many other dietitians contributed with ideas and tried out the practical aspects of the study and for weeks telephone calls and letters were flying up and down the country whilst the study was developed.

This was the first time a study of this kind had been attempted and at this stage no one quite realised how big it was going to turn out to be. Although many nutrition surveys have been done, none have been conducted with the expertise of dietitians being used to investigate the practicality of people changing their eating habits.

What we tried to do

1 Find out what, if any, obstacles and problems dietitians and adult members of their households experienced when trying to eat a diet which conforms to the long-term nutritional guidelines recommended by NACNE. This could be achieved by:

- establishing how many participants were already eating a diet achieving the long-term guidelines
- establishing how nearly the long-term nutritional guidelines could be attained by the participants
- finding out the effect of dietary changes on the lifestyles of the participants

2 Provide information from which to devise guidelines on

suitable types of foods and meal patterns required to achieve the nutritional guidelines which can be used as the basis for advice to the general public. This could be achieved by:
- identifying individuals who achieved the long-term guidelines
- collecting information from the food diaries of these individuals

3 To test the feasibility of the survey methods for use on a larger population sample drawn from the general public.

How we did it

We enrolled dietitians, their spouses, friends and relatives via an advertisement in the BDA's newsletter. They were then asked to keep a detailed record for one week while eating as they usually did. Next they were asked to change their pattern of eating so as to conform as far as possible to the long-term NACNE goals and to keep a record for a second week. In a sense this was tough because we were asking them to achieve 'overnight' what NACNE said should be done over 15 years!

The participants in the study were thus a self-selected group of dietitians and adult members of their households who replied to notices in the newsletter sent to them from the BDA office or in the CNG correspondence. (Children were not included in the study because the guidelines suggested by NACNE are directly applicable to adults. It was hoped that as many men as possible would participate because they would have higher daily energy requirements and, being mainly non-dietitians, might be less motivated to change their eating patterns.

The target was to attract a minimum of 100 people for the study. The response was far above this. This highlighted the importance dietitians were giving to it – especially when they knew of the extra work they were letting themselves in for! Over 500 people volunteered to join the survey and finally 472 people were involved.

Participants were asked to record two separate seven-day weighed food intakes of everything they ate and drank both at home and outside. They also had to answer brief questionnaires about how changes in their eating habits had affected their lifestyles.

The first food diary was to be kept whilst eating as normally as possible and the dietary analysis of this was to be used as a basis for change. Brief written advice was given to each individual and then the dietitian participants were asked to use their own expertise to effect these changes. Non-dietitians were to seek advice from the dietitian in their household.

The Timetable of the Study

A letter outlining the study and calling for volunteers was issued in a CNG mailing and published in the BDA's Newsletter.

Applicants were then sent a food diary which had a code number differentiating between dietitians and non-dietitians, male and female. An accompanying letter gave instructions on how to complete the week's food survey.

Participants who did not return their food diaries within this time were telephoned and asked to return them, completed, within a further two weeks. If they still failed to do so they were sent a letter asking for their reasons, together with a stamped addressed envelope to return the uncompleted diary to the project team.

The food diaries and questionnaires were then coded for computer analysis by dietitians and coordinated by the research dietitian at the Institute of Zoology in London. These were analysed by the programmer of the Nuffield Laboratories at the Institute. The Institute of Zoology is more affectionately referred to as the 'Zoo' and this set many participants to wondering exactly what sort of study they were involved in! Examples of the two computer print-outs sent to the participants are given in the Appendix at the end of the book and show just how detailed the food analyses and advice were.

The participants whose food intakes achieved all the long-term guidelines during the first week of recording had their analyses returned to them with a letter thanking them for their help and cooperation. Less formally their diaries were likely to be marked BINGO! as the project team were delighted to see the NACNE guidelines being met whilst the participants were 'eating normally'. A second questionnaire was also sent which found out whether the 'first time achievers' had changed their eating habits over the last two years or more.

The participants who did not achieve all of the long-term guidelines whilst they were eating normally were then sent a copy of the analysis of their first week's food intake (an example is shown in the Appendix) with a letter asking them to make a determined effort to change their eating habits during this second week to meet the long-term guidelines. Once again detailed instructions were given inside the food diaries and a lot of emphasis was put on the accurate recording of data. It was assumed that all the dietitian participants would have recorded their food intake at some time in the past (perhaps as a part of their training) and that the non-dietitians were unlikely ever to have done so. Weighing foods at home for most people started as a novelty but this soon wore off when dinner was seen to be getting cold. Weighing food in a canteen or restaurant certainly caused hilarity for some participants and embarrassment to others as it is a somewhat unusual pastime. When weighing things at home the dietitian in the house was called upon to ensure an accurate description of all the foods.

The food diary also contained detailed instructions about the measurements to record and other general information to be recorded, for example where foods were eaten, to help monitor any changes in lifestyle which might be made during the survey. Participants were asked on their questionnaire at the end of the first week whether 'they thought that the weighing and recording of their food intake altered their normal eating habits during the survey'. Most of the participants thought that it had not affected their normal eating but those who thought it had said that although they had tried hard not to let it the tendency had been to eat fewer second helpings, fewer snacks, to nibble less often and not to eat the children's leftovers. People also found that they simplified recipes to save weighing and recording ingredients. A participant who was very close to achieving the long-term guidelines on her first attempt commented that 'being in the survey and thinking of food increased the amount of food I ate.'

A questionnaire, reproduced in the Appendix, was completed at the end of the second week to help identify any changes which might have been made in the participants' lifestyles. Three weeks was the time allocated for this and people were followed up if they were late in returning them to the project team.

Returned food diaries and questionnaires were coded and analysed, as in the first instance. The results (see Appendix for an example) were sent back to participants with a letter of thanks for their help and cooperation.

The participants were more than pleased, after the survey week, to be able to sit to a meal or eat a snack which did not have to be weighed or described.

The findings of the study are reported in Chapter 3 but there is one question taken from questionnaire 1 which is relevant here. It is the response to the question 'Do you agree with setting dietary goals for a population?' Most of the participants, whether dietitians or not, replied 'yes' to this question and many made additional comments which can be summarised into four points:

- Most people wanted to see general *guidelines* for the population rather than strict goals.
- Many participants stressed that these should not only be for the general public but also for the Government and the food industry.
- Having guidelines was seen to be essential for providing a basis from which educational programmes could be devised whilst ensuring consistent information throughout the country.
- The nutritional guidelines needed to be translated into terms of foods, meal plans and recipes for the general population.

For more of the individual participants' thoughts on this subject, see Chapter 4.

The final part of the Study took the form of in-depth group interviews in four major centres at which a total of 10 per cent of all the participants completing the two-week study were gathered. This feature was not originally planned as part of the study but it became apparent that the participants had a lot to say that could not easily be recorded on the questionnaires. Given that the participants were mainly trained professionals, whose opinions could (and indeed should) be of value, we decided to obtain them at a formal, yet relaxed, interview and then present them as part of the book. The results of these interviews form the basis for Chapter 4.

CHAPTER THREE

The Results of the Study

Who Took Part?

As we saw in Chapter 2, 472 adults took part in the study; 304 women and 168 men. Most of the women were dietitians. In all there were 289 dietitians and 183 non-dietitians.

The participants came from all over the United Kingdom; the majority were aged between 20 and 40, and most were white, professional workers. Physical activity levels varied but most claimed to be moderately active. The vast majority were meat eaters although a handful were vegetarians.

The majority, 84 per cent, said that they agreed with the concept of setting dietary guidelines for the population. The group was, therefore, motivated to put the NACNE nutritional guidelines to the test.

Trying to Achieve the NACNE Goals

Each specific NACNE goal is not for individuals nor for sub-groups of the population, such as groups of men, women and children. It was, however, necessary in this study to apply the goals to individuals in order to classify them as 'achieving', 'very close to achieving' and 'not quite achieving'. After all, the changes will in reality have to be made by individuals and families. The division of the group in this way was to help identify food choices and habits that are in line with the healthier way of eating.

The 'achieving group' included both those individuals who

actually achieved the full six NACNE goals, and those coming within a 10 per cent margin of all the goals. This group was nicknamed YES. The 'very close to achieving' group were those that fell just outside the 10 per cent margin for one goal – these were termed NEAR. The rest of the group, the 'not quite NACNE' individuals we called NO.

Interpreting the Goals

In order to apply NACNE recommendations to individuals for this study a certain degree of interpretation of the goals had to take place.

The total fat, saturated fat and fibre goals could be interpreted from NACNE without any modification. All the individuals were asked to achieve the same goal of 30g fibre. This was done in spite of the fact that it is easier for people who eat more calories to achieve the fibre goal. It was felt better not to pre-judge this issue but to find out more about this link from the study.

The remaining three goals of sugar, salt and alcohol needed further dietetic interpretation.

In the NACNE Report the long-term goal for sugar is 20kg/head/year. This refers to the most commonly used type of sugar, sucrose. Other types of sugar can also be added (e.g. glucose, corn syrup solids). The sugar analysed from foods in this study was the total added sugars from selected foods, such as cakes, biscuits, sugary drinks, jams and sweets. When all the sugars are included, this provides nearly 20 per cent of total calories. Therefore a figure of 10 per cent of total calories from added sugar was used as a maximum for this goal.

The NACNE long-term goal for salt is a recommended reduction from the present consumption. Pilot attempts at weighing salt added when cooking at home and at meal times were unsuccessful, therefore only the salt already in food was analysed. Even this analysis was an underestimate as the salt added to dishes cooked in restaurants, cafés and canteens could not be allowed for. The 9g salt goal in the study was therefore more lenient than that included in NACNE. All the participants were asked whether they added salt to their food and those who did and who also had a level near the goal, were advised to reduce their intake.

The long-term goal of 4 per cent of total calories from alcohol given by NACNE is an average for the population and will therefore include non-drinkers. Individual drinkers are not necessarily expected to keep within the 4 per cent level. A figure of 8 per cent of calories from alcohol was taken as the upper limit for individuals, based on a World Health Organisation publication. The 4 per cent level was applied when looking at all our participants as a group. This level is quite strict as it was a purely adult group, not including any children who are non-drinkers and help to bring the average level down.

NACNE also set short-term goals for the 1980s. Short-term goals were interpreted from NACNE in the same way as the long-term ones.

Summary of the Goals Used in the Study for Individuals

	Long-term goals	Short-term goals
fat%*	30	34
saturated fat%*	10	15
added sugar%*	10	12
alcohol%*	8†(4)	(5)
fibre g	30	25
sodium (salt) mg	3600	4300

*percentage of calories consumed
( )this is the average applied to the group
†this is the level applied for individuals

The Participants' Normal Diet (The First Week)

All the participants ate their normal everyday foods when completing the first week's weighed food intake. How did the group's normal diet compare with the goals?

Comparison of the Participants' Normal Diet with the Study's Goals (472 participants)

Dietary component	BDA study results	Long-term goal*	Short-term goal*	Present average for the whole population (ref: NACNE)
fat%†	36	30	34	38
saturated fat%†	14	10	15	18
added sugar%†	8	10	16	18‡
alcohol%†	5	4	5	6
fibre g	29	30	25	20
sodium mg	2879	3600	4300	4700

*interpreted from NACNE
†percentage of calories consumed
‡(sources: *Towards a Sugar Health Policy* and *The Food Scandal* (see page 242)

Better Than the Average Diet
The dietitians and those they influenced in the study were already eating a diet nearly in line with the short-term goals so on the whole they practise what they preach. The fat was slightly high but the sugar intake was well below the long-term goal. The message to reduce sugar in the interest of better teeth and weight control has been prominent for years, allowing people to interpret and adopt low-sugar food choices. The message to reduce fat is relatively recent.

The Second Week

What happened when participants completed their second diaries and were trying to alter their eating habits in the direction of the long-term goals? There were 351 people who completed this second week (209 women and 142 men).

Comparison of Second Diaries with Long-term Goals (351 Participants)

Dietary component	BDA study results	Long-term goals
fat%*	30	30
saturated fat%*	10	10
added sugar%*	7	10
alcohol%*	4	4
fibre g	38	30
sodium mg	2691	3600

*percentage of calories consumed

Success!

The group as a whole achieved these goals in spite of the fact that a time span of 15 years had been given to achieve the goals by gradual changes. The participants had to make changes almost overnight. It should be noted that while 47 per cent were able to give a confident 'yes' to the healthy eating pattern becoming a permanent way of life, a further 27 per cent were uncertain about continuing and 26 per cent felt that they couldn't maintain the necessary changes. One participant's only comment was 'less bran, more ale!'

The main obstacles to maintaining this type of diet included:

missing certain foods, such as sweets, snacks, chips, fat and dairy products
extra time required in preparing basic foods
lack of suitable foods available at work and in restaurants
lack of suitable convenience foods
lack of suitable snacks to eat in between meals
the bulk of the diet

Let us now look at the progress of individuals to find out more about each of the goals, the foods and habits associated with achieving and not achieving the goals, and other nutritional aspects of the healthier diets.

Individuals Completing the First Diary

The Results of the First Week (472 Participants)

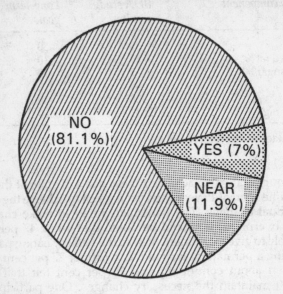

When considering individuals, most people did not achieve all the long-term goals. However, 33 participants were already eating a diet within 10 per cent of the goals, with women more successful than men. This is perhaps to be expected as the majority of the women were dietitians.

So how did individuals get on when trying to eat differently in the NACNE style? Those already eating according to the goals did not complete a second diary.

Individuals Completing the Second Diary

The Results of the Second Week (351 Participants)

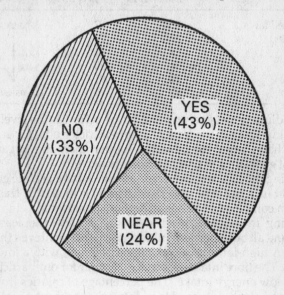

This time more participants were in the YES group where all six goals were achieved, than in the NO group who had clearly fallen short of the goals. Again women fared better than men.

Which Goals Were the Hardest to Achieve?

The next table indicates that the saturated fat and the total fat goals proved to be the hardest and required the greatest effort on the part of the participants. This is not surprising when we consider the fact that so much of our fat is in a hidden form in food. The amount of fat in food is to a large extent decided for us.

Percentage of Participants who Achieved Specific Goals

	First week (% of 472)	Second week (% of 351)	
Saturated fat	17	67	hardest
Total fat	27	71	
Fibre	53	81	
Sugar	81	90	↓
Alcohol	81	91	
Sodium	92	95	easiest

The sodium or salt goal appeared to be easiest as the level set in the study was on the lenient side. A stricter goal for sodium could have been considerably harder than the sugar and alcohol goals for the participants to achieve.

During the first week everyone achieved at least one goal; in fact all but 1 per cent (five participants) achieved at least two goals, a combination of sugar, sodium or alcohol.

During the second week everyone achieved at least two goals and all but 3 per cent (nine participants) achieved three or more. A high fat intake was often combined with a low fibre intake. The fibre intake was indeed harder for our participants with a low energy intake. The percentage of calories from fat, sugar and alcohol seemed to be interrelated where a high level of one tended to push down the others.

Calorie (Energy) Intake

One of the significant findings of this study was the effect that the effort to achieve the goals had on energy or calorie intake.

Average Energy Intake in Calories

	First week	Second week	Recommended daily allowance (RDA)
Women	(n = 304) 1893	(n = 209) 1688	2150
Men	(n = 168) 2591	(n = 142) 2251	2900

n = number of participants

The initial intake of the group as a whole was well below that recommended by the DHSS. In the 'Recommended Daily Allowance of Food Energy and Nutrients in the UK' (RDA) it recommends specific amounts of food energy and nutrients for healthy groups of people living in the UK. It was found that almost everyone had decreased their calorie intake in the second diaries. The average was a drop of 11 per cent. Also the average energy intake for those who achieved was lower than for those who did not.

The calorie intake varied considerably between individuals and in fact the highest and lowest intakes both came from people who did not achieve all the goals.

It is worth mentioning that the researchers had expected a drop in energy intake when participants tried to achieve the goals. They had therefore asked all the participants to try hard to maintain their energy intake. The drop in energy intake can be explained as follows:

As starchy food is bulky (you need, for example, to eat one slice of wholemeal bread to get as many calories as you get from a small pat of butter), someone who is not used to the bulk can find it difficult to eat enough. It would be easier if more in-between meal snacks were eaten, but at the moment there are very few snack foods available which are low in fat, salt and sugar yet high in fibre. A combination of this lack of availability of suitable snacks and feelings of fullness stopped many of our participants from eating between meals, even when they had previously done so. This resulted in the fall in their calorie intake. We had, after all, asked the participants to do overnight what NACNE asked the population to do in 15 years.

Do People Adapt to the NACNE Way of Eating?

In short – yes, people do to some extent adapt to more bulk. The participants who achieved all the goals when eating normally were compared with the group who achieved all the goals when doing the second diary.

Average Energy Intakes in Calories for the YES Group

	First week	Second week
Women	(n = 30) 1829	(n = 102) 1673

n = number of participants

The women achieving on the first diary were eating more than those making an effort to reach NACNE the second time. A similar comparison cannot be made for the men as the number of achievers in the first week is too small. It would seem that those who choose to follow the NACNE style of eating must find ways of eating more food. There seem to be three lessons to be learned from these particular results:

- Sudden, dramatic changes, such as those made by the participants in this study, could not be maintained for long. The body needs time to adjust to the increased bulk. Gradual changes are more likely to be long-lasting.
- To eat the extra bulk called for by a more healthy diet it may be necessary for some people to eat more in between meal snacks as well as more for meals.
- There is a need for snack foods, low in fat and sugar and high in fibre from food manufacturers, canteens and cafés.

The question may be raised as to why all the participants, both those achieving and not achieving, had energy intakes so far below the Recommended Daily Amounts. One reason could be that the recommended amounts are too high for our current lifestyles. Another reason could be that weighing and recording everything eaten for a week is enough to decrease most people's appetite. 'I don't feel like a biscuit thank you – I'm far too comfortable in my chair to go and find the weighing scales, diary and a pen!' The participants were asked whether the weighing and recording of the food had an effect on their eating patterns:

62 per cent felt they had not changed the way they ate for that week

30 per cent felt they had
8 per cent were uncertain.

The weighing of the food may have influenced the group's eating habits to some extent.

What Effect did the NACNE Way of Eating have on Other Nutrients in the Diet?

The majority of nutrients increased on the NACNE-style diet, despite the drop in calorie intakes. If calorie levels had been maintained when achieving the goals, the increase in nutrients might have been even greater. The NACNE-style diet is therefore richer in most nutrients than our participants' normal diets.

Nutrient Intakes Significantly Different Between the YES and NO Groups

MEN

Nutrient	NO group	YES group	RDA
Iron mg	18	21	10
Zinc mg	13.3	14.7	15*
Niacin (Vit B$_3$) mg	45	48	18
Vitamin C mg	107	135	30
Vitamin E mg	9.7	11.5	15*
Vitamin B$_6$ mg	1.9	2.3	2*
Folic Acid mcg	274	323	300

WOMEN

Nutrient	NO group	YES group	RDA
Iron mg	15	18	12
Zinc mg	10.6	12.2	15*
Vitamin D mcg	3.6	4.3	Sunlight†
Niacin (Vit B$_3$) mg	35	38	15
Vitamin C mg	104	126	30

WOMEN – *continued*

Nutrient	NO group	YES group	RDA
Vitamin E mg	7.5	8.7	12*
Vitamin B_6 mg	1.5	2.0	2*
Folic Acid mcg	225	277	300

*USA recommendations have been used as there are no British recommendations for these nutrients.
†No specific recommendation is made – sunlight is the main source of Vitamin D.
RDA Recommended Daily Amount

Protein, calcium, Vitamin A (and in the case of men, Vitamin D), riboflavin and Vitamin B_{12} were not significantly different between the two groups, but all were well above the RDA. Some participants failed to reach the RDAs for certain nutrients. Fifty eight women (19 per cent) did not achieve the RDA for iron in the first week. Of these, 52 failed to achieve the goals as well. In the second week, when a definite attempt was made to improve diets, only 23 women (11 per cent) were low in iron intake. Again the majority, 18 of them, were in the NO group.

Achieving the dietary goals tends to make the diet more 'nutrient-dense'. It has been shown that this style of eating is not likely to result in mineral or vitamin deficiencies, as some critics have proposed.

Types of Food Making up the Diets of the YES and NO Groups

Having looked at the overall diet eaten by the participants achieving the long-term goals we can examine the types of foods which they ate. As we have one section which achieved the goals and one which did not it is possible to compare the foods eaten by each group.

There were many differences between them. The table on pages 48 and 49 shows how the YES group's diet differed from that of the NO group: taking the NO group as the base the chart shows how much more (or less) of a particular food the YES group ate.

The YES group ate more of the foods on the right, and less of the foods on the left, than the NO group. How much more or less is indicated in the brackets.

From the differences it is interesting to look in more detail at the types of foods eaten by each of these groups. When comparing the two diets we must remember that we are looking at the *average* amounts of foods eaten by these two 'populations'. The average includes everybody, whether or not they ate a particular food. The individual diets contributing to that average varied greatly. (The emphasis of this study is on the eating patterns of populations rather than individuals). Thus we can see interesting differences in the food choices made by the achieving and non-achieving groups but not of any one individual.

There is no such thing as a 'perfect diet' as many combinations of foods will achieve the dietary goals. Therefore the quantities of foods which will now be discussed show only the types and amounts of foods eaten by the two groups. In Chapter 5 you will then find more ideas and suggestions which will help you choose a diet you enjoy.

Consumption of Cereal Foods

The YES group ate more cereals, bread (especially wholemeal), pasta, rice and fewer biscuits, cakes, pastries and puddings than the NO group. This helps to explain why some people found their diet to be bulkier than usual. The table on page 50 shows the amounts of some of these foods eaten.

Overleaf: the diagrammatic representation of how the YES group's diet differed from that of the NO group.

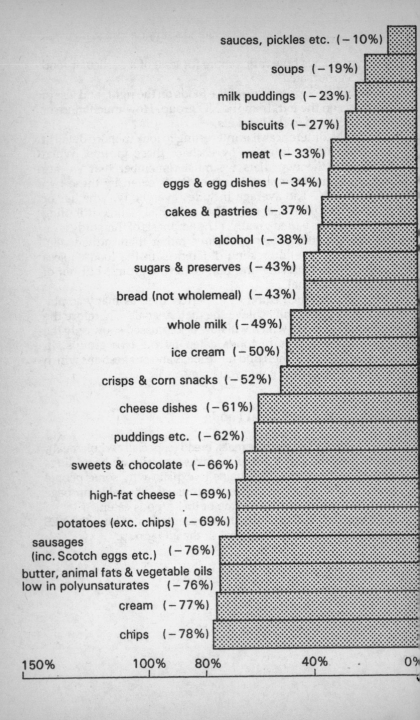

sauces, pickles etc. (−10%)

soups (−19%)

milk puddings (−23%)

biscuits (−27%)

meat (−33%)

eggs & egg dishes (−34%)

cakes & pastries (−37%)

alcohol (−38%)

sugars & preserves (−43%)

bread (not wholemeal) (−43%)

whole milk (−49%)

ice cream (−50%)

crisps & corn snacks (−52%)

cheese dishes (−61%)

puddings etc. (−62%)

sweets & chocolate (−66%)

high-fat cheese (−69%)

potatoes (exc. chips) (−69%)

sausages (inc. Scotch eggs etc.) (−76%)

butter, animal fats & vegetable oils low in polyunsaturates (−76%)

cream (−77%)

chips (−78%)

150%   100%   80%   40%   0%

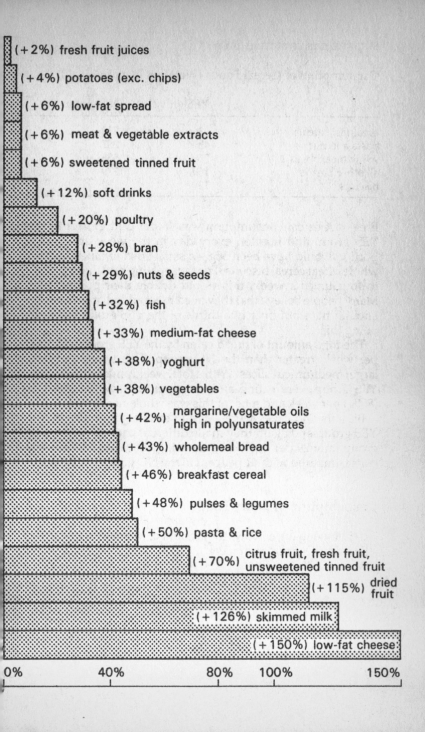

(+2%) fresh fruit juices

(+4%) potatoes (exc. chips)

(+6%) low-fat spread

(+6%) meat & vegetable extracts

(+6%) sweetened tinned fruit

(+12%) soft drinks

(+20%) poultry

(+28%) bran

(+29%) nuts & seeds

(+32%) fish

(+33%) medium-fat cheese

(+38%) yoghurt

(+38%) vegetables

(+42%) margarine/vegetable oils high in polyunsaturates

(+43%) wholemeal bread

(+46%) breakfast cereal

(+48%) pulses & legumes

(+50%) pasta & rice

(+70%) citrus fruit, fresh fruit, unsweetened tinned fruit

(+115%) dried fruit

(+126%) skimmed milk

(+150%) low-fat cheese

0%   40%   80%   100%   150%

Consumption of Cereal Foods (Weighed in g per Week)

	YES group	NO group
breakfast cereals	336	230
pasta and rice	430	287
wholemeal bread	760	533
all other breads	160	279
biscuits	138	190

Breakfast cereal consumption was 46 per cent greater in the YES group and if eaten every day in the week an average portion would have been 50g – a small bowl of muesli or two wholewheat cereal biscuits. For those eating cereals only three to four times a week, this would double their portion size. Many people believe that they need to eat added bran to obtain enough fibre but over two-thirds of the YES group were not doing this.

The total amount of bread eaten by the YES group was 100g per week greater than the NO group. This would be three large, medium-cut slices. With a total weekly intake of 920g the YES group were eating an average of just over a large loaf (800g) per week and most of this was wholemeal bread.

Biscuits and cakes were eaten in smaller quantities by the YES group and again they made different choices. In the YES group only 29 per cent were choosing chocolate-covered biscuits compared with 41 per cent in the NO group.

Consumption of Dairy Foods

The following table shows the amount of milk consumed in the YES and NO groups per week.

Consumption of Milk (Pints per Week)

	YES group	NO group
milk – whole	1.1	2.1
milk – skimmed	2.2	1.0
milk – semi-skimmed	0.03	0.03
Total	3.33	3.13

A clear difference in choice is seen as both groups had an average of just over 3 pints milk for each individual per week. However the YES group were having over two of these as skimmed milk. Interestingly there was no difference in the intake of semi-skimmed milk and this was a very small proportion of the total.

Looking at other dairy foods, a similar trend can again be seen with lower-fat products being consumed to a greater extent by the YES group.

Consumption of Other Dairy Foods (g per Week)

	YES group	NO group
yoghurt	225	163
cream	6	26
low-fat cheese	158	63
medium-fat cheese	28	21
high-fat cheese	47	152

As a population the YES group ate on average 6g of cream each during one week but only 18 per cent of the group actually ate cream. For those 18 per cent their intake ranged from 5 to 100g. This highlights the point that individuals within the group were able to include some high-fat foods depending on their other food choices.

However, if we take the populations as a whole we find that the YES group would have been eating approximately one quarter of the cream eaten by the NO group and 6g of cream is little more than one teaspoon.

Both the YES and NO groups ate about 230g cheese per week (or just over 8oz) in total. Again the types of cheeses which were consumed differed between the two groups. The YES group were eating mainly low-fat cheese, like cottage cheese and skimmed milk cheese, whilst the NO group ate mainly higher-fat cheeses such as hard English cheeses and soft 'cream' cheeses.

Cheese and egg dishes and eggs were also eaten in smaller quantities by the YES group as were ice cream and milk puddings. Let us look only at those people who ate ice cream. In the YES group their average intake was 43g (less than a 50g or 2oz scoop) yet in the NO group they ate an average of 147g (3 scoops) per week.

We can see then that as a population whilst the same foods are being chosen by both groups the YES group were either choosing lower-fat alternatives, when available, or having smaller portions.

Consumption of Meat and Fish

Consumption of Meat and Fish (g per Week)

	YES group	NO group
all meats	310	464
poultry	188	157
meat products (including sausages)	52	185
all fish	247	187

Comparing the two populations we again see the trends of the YES group eating smaller quantities of the high-fat products such as sausages and meat products and more of the less fatty foods such as poultry and fish. As a population the NO group ate over three times as much of the meat products as the NO group.

Looking only at the people who ate poultry, then the average portion chosen by the YES group was 16 per cent larger than that of the NO group.

Thus within these foods a similar situation is found to that of the choice of dairy foods.

Consumption of Pulse Vegetables

Pulse vegetables, beans and lentils, can be served either as a side vegetable or as a main dish. When used as a main dish they are often chosen as an alternative to animal protein foods such as red meats and cheese, giving a protein source which is low in fat and containing fibre. It is particularly interesting to look at the quantities eaten by the YES and NO groups and the proportions of each population eating them.

In the YES group 99.5 per cent of the group ate an average of 455g (16oz) per week cooked weights compared to 80 per cent of the NO group having an average weekly consumption of 382g (13½oz). Once again, this shows the characteristics of the populations as a whole and not individual consumption. There was a wide range of consumption for those individuals eating pulses in the YES group from 10 to 1100g. The person with the highest intake was also eating a small amount of meat and fish so was not a vegetarian.

In Chapter 5 you will find more information about the variety of beans that are available which can add new dimensions to your meals.

Consumption of Potatoes, Root, Green and Salad Vegetables

This table shows the average weekly consumption of the total YES and NO groups.

Consumption of Vegetables (g per Week)

	YES group	NO group
potatoes	580	559
chips	19	87
crisps	11	23
all vegetables (excluding potatoes) and salad	1564	1132

The YES group as an average ate 432g (nearly 1lb) more a week of all vegetables and salad vegetables (excluding potatoes) than the NO group. (The weights shown are the actual weights consumed, not the weights prior to preparation.)

If we look at potatoes, excluding chips and crisps there is no difference between the YES and NO groups.

Although in both groups less than 1 in 5 ate chips the consumption was nearly four times as high in the NO group.

In the YES group the individual recording the lowest weekly consumption of chips, at 25g, possibly took about 3 chips from someone else's plate!

Consumption of Fruit, Nuts and Seeds

The following table shows the average weekly consumption of these foods for the YES and NO groups as a whole.

Consumption of Fruit, Nuts and Seeds (g per week)

	YES group	NO group
fresh & unsweetened fruit	1810	1067
fruit juice	271	265
dried fruits	56	26
nuts & seeds	49	38

The YES group ate over one and a half times as much fruit. They also ate more dried fruit, nuts and seeds.

Consumption of Sugar and Sweets

Consumption of Sugar and Sweets (g per week)

	YES group	NO group
sugar & preserves	59	105
sweets	21	62

We have seen earlier in this chapter that the participants met the long-term goal for sugar whilst eating their normal diet. Here we can see the difference in sugar consumption for the YES and NO groups and find that on average the YES group ate 59g (2oz) of sugar and preserves per week compared to 105g (nearly 4oz) in the NO group. In the YES group 82.5 per cent of the population were eating added sugar and/or preserves with a weekly intake ranging from 5–319g amongst these individuals.

Consumption of Fats for Spreading and Cooking

Consumption of Fats (g per week)

	YES group	NO group
total spreading fats	145	188
total cooking oils and fats	48	81
total fats	193	269

As expected the YES group were eating less total fat than the NO group. If we break this down into the types of fats used the table below shows the lower intake of saturated fats and greater intake of polyunsaturated fats for the YES group when compared to the NO group.

Types of Fats Used (g)

	YES group	NO group
total fats and oils high in saturated fat	34	141
total fats and oils high in polyunsaturates	91	64
total low-fat spreads	68	64

Can we gain an idea of the amount and types of fat people within the YES group were buying? The YES group used an average of about 145g of spreading fats each per week of which about 65g were polyunsaturates and 72g were low-fat spreads. As a group the total amount of butter and other margarines was less than 15g per week.

Despite the fact that some people chose low-fat spreads, their fat intake from spreading fats was similar to that of those choosing full-fat products due to the fact they used nearly double the amount. They were therefore paying twice as much for the same amount of fat.

If we look at cooking fats the YES group on average were using just under 50g per week, most of which were oils high in polyunsaturates.

Consumption of Alcohol

When looking at alcohol consumption, we have already given reasons for taking an upper limit of 8 per cent of total energy intake as the long-term goal in this study. Both the YES and NO groups were well within this limit, having an average intake of 3.3 per cent and 4.8 per cent of energy from alcohol respectively.

To translate this into more readily accepted terms, we have

chosen to use the system of alcohol units as used by the Health Education Council.

1 unit of alcohol is equivalent to:

½ pint beer
1 glass wine
1 measure (⅙ gill) spirits.

For the YES group 3.3 per cent of their combined daily energy intake (for men and women) gives an average of 1 unit of alcohol per day or 7 units per week. For the NO group the figure is closer to 1½ units per day or 10 units per week.

The Effects on Lifestyle

Having seen that the participants as a group were able to achieve the long-term dietary goals, it is important to consider the trials and tribulations that went into accomplishing this. Participants were asked to complete extensive questionnaires to monitor the effect that the changes in food choices had on aspects of their lifestyles during the study week, and how they felt about the changes that they were making.

As the entire group were asked to make the same sorts of changes, everyone's responses are considered together, as well as noting particular differences between the YES group and the NO group. These differences can point out and help to explain the specific areas that helped or hindered our participants in their attempts to change their diets.

Did People Enjoy Their Food?

This is perhaps one of the most important questions we asked the participants during the study week. Without meeting this essential criterion, it is doubtful whether any change, even for the benefits of better health, would be maintained. As a group 62 per cent said they enjoyed their food just as much as usual, 10 per cent said more, but 28 per cent said less. This was similar for those who did and did not achieve the goals.

When asked if there were any factors that limited the enjoyment of their food, 55 per cent of the group said 'yes'. Besides two responses of 'Yes, my wife is a dietitian!' the most frequently mentioned factors included:

the extra time required for planning, shopping and preparation of food

the lack of availability and variety of suitable foods, particularly convenience foods

the increased cost, although when asked about cost in the next question, very few stated that they had spent more on food.

leaving out favourite foods felt to be unhealthy (such as cheese, biscuits and chocolate) and guilt felt if they were eaten.

A small number of those failing to achieve the goals, but none in the achieving group, stated that a lack of knowledge about which foods to choose limited their enjoyment. This supports the need to translate dietary goals expressed as percentages and grams into clear dietary guidelines based on types and amounts of foods.

Did Food Cost Any More?

When asked the question 'Do you think the amount you spent on food was more, the same, or less than usual?' the majority of the group, 67 per cent, said the same, 12 per cent said less, and 21 per cent said more. It is interesting to note that only 10 per cent more in the YES group than the NO group stated that they had spent more on food. Therefore cost can be a concern, but need not be a major hurdle, in choosing a healthier diet.

Did it Take Longer to Prepare Food?

The participants were asked to give an estimate of the amount of time they spent each day preparing food. Half the people felt they had spent more time when preparing the NACNE-style food. This may be the result of a shortage of convenience foods compatible with NACNE. As a result, people spent a similar amount of money but more time preparing healthy but less quick-to-prepare foods from basic ingredients:

54 per cent said they had spent more time
11 per cent said they had spent less time
35 per cent said they spent the same amount of time as usual.

The most common food preparation time when attempting to change to healthier foods was between one and two hours. Fifty two per cent of the YES group spent this amount of time, compared to 40 per cent of the NO group. More striking is the fact that 21 per cent of those who failed to reach the goals spent less than half an hour preparing food, compared to 7 per cent for the YES group, and may reflect the use of convenience foods. There was no difference between these groups for those reporting more than two hours preparing food.

Did you Change Recipes, Ingredients or Cooking Methods?

Participants were asked if they deliberately used different recipes or ingredients or altered their cooking methods in order to achieve the goals.

More people (85 per cent) who achieved the goals said that they did change their recipes and ingredients as compared to those who did not achieve the goals (70 per cent). Only 40 per cent of the group altered their cooking methods; this is true for both the YES and NO groups.

How did Your Efforts Affect Your Shopping?

Participants were asked to record where they did their shopping, in order of frequency. This was to find out if they needed to use different shops to meet the goals.

Although some people found they had to make changes in their shop choices, most (79 per cent) did not. The YES group were less likely to use different shops (26 per cent) than were the NO group (57 per cent). Further, the NO group were as likely to choose a traditional shop as they were a wholefood or health food shop, perhaps a factor in their ultimate results.

The effort of shopping for healthier foods was noted by more people in the YES group (39 per cent) than the NO group (25 per cent). This shows that decisions made when shopping are seen to have a bearing on overall chances of eating a healthier diet.

Supermarkets claimed the trade of 82 per cent of the group as a first preferred choice. Second and third choices of shops varied considerably, but taken together, the following shops were used:

56 per cent used traditional shops such as butchers, bakers and greengrocers
34 per cent used markets
30 per cent used small general stores
28 per cent used health food and wholefood shops.

Did Other Members of the Family Eat Meals Similar to Yours?

On the whole, there were no differences between the YES and NO group, the household ate the same sort of food as the participants – 85 per cent said they did, 15 per cent did not. Where different meals were eaten these were primarily lunches eaten outside the home and meals prepared for small children or difficult husbands!

Did Attempting to Change your Food Pattern Affect your Social Activities?

A major problem for 37 per cent of the group was curtailing social activities whereas 63 per cent claimed generally to maintain their normal social activities.

A quarter of the group (27 per cent) said they ate less in

restaurants in an attempt to achieve the goals. It was found that 13 per cent of the NO group claimed to eat in restaurants more often this week. As this was not found in the YES group, it might be assumed that present restaurant choices are less conducive to the low-sugar/fat/salt, high-fibre way of eating. As the number of meals eaten away from home is steadily increasing, restaurant food must be considered when recommending changes on a national level.

Were you Able to Use the Office or Works Canteen?

When asked about the frequency of eating in the office or works canteen, more of the YES group (35 per cent) reported eating fewer meals prepared at work than the NO group (19 per cent). Although the majority were maintaining their use of office and works catering facilities, again the role of these outlets in providing suitable foods is important. As time is already a concern, more time spent preparing suitable lunches to take to work is not a welcome addition to the day!

CHAPTER FOUR

What the Participants Had to Say

Of those who completed the second week's part of the study we interviewed 40 face to face in small groups. It was during this part of the study that the dietitians and their families came across as real human beings with the same problems as other people when it comes to changing their eating habits.

Only 7 per cent of the participants were eating according to the NACNE guidelines during the first study week but this went up to 43 per cent second time around, so obviously they were making a very real effort. Remember when reading this chapter that we were asking people to make changes to a NACNE diet over a very short period of time. The NACNE recommendations allowed years for such changes to happen (see page 10). Also, we were asking each individual to achieve every goal whereas NACNE asks the whole population to achieve it on average. Individuals for example who drink no alcohol and eat little sugar naturally find the fat goal harder. People who need a lot of calories find the salt goal hard to achieve. Even so, it shows what can be done, even if with some difficulty, given the sharp changes required in the buying, preparation and eating of food.

Question 1: What are Your Overall Impressions of Doing the Study?

Clearly, people's answers varied enormously according to their personalities and how much the whole thing had impressed them as a way of eating for the future. Please note that the following quotations show some of the personal views and thoughts that our participants had and may not reflect overall views or the views of the authors.

'I was quite surprised when I got my first week back as I had a lot more fibre than I actually thought I had. When I got to the second week I was just having to cut down the fat, which I did by just using skimmed milk and cottage cheese and yoghurt. I used as much margarine, and I still made crumbles and things. And I got it down to the NACNE recommendations. Alcohol is not a problem. I found snacks very difficult. I was hungry all the time. I could not stick to eating that way all the time. I could do it for most of the time, but I would still like to have some double cream and things.'

'I was surprised how bad my diet was in the first place. I did not find it difficult to cut my fat or sugar. But my boyfriend found it really hard. It was difficult to find substitutes for sandwich fillings without having cheese etc. Also he is underweight with a small appetite so with cutting the fat he found it very difficult to keep his calories up. He felt he was eating non-stop all day.'

'Healthy snacks are the biggest problem. I didn't want more fruit, I didn't want more bread and I didn't want more cereal. I was already having six or seven slices of bread a day and big bowls of cereals, and I didn't want more.'

'I think the big problem people have about going to a NACNE-type diet is that they always try to cut out things. But looking at it from the other way is what can you add. Because my calorie intake is 2700 that is why I could get away with so much sugar. Rather than saying, "What could I substitute for high-fat things?" it was more a case of looking from the Continental way of just starting off with the basic cereal or staple kind of thing to which all the other fatty things are just the trimmings. That way there was never the problem about having enough to eat, nor was there a problem of cutting out, it was a question of putting in.'

'I can now taste the salt that is in bread and I found the amount of salt which one actually buys in bought foods makes it difficult to attune your taste buds. My cooking is salt-free, and I have found plenty of alternatives to salt to use in cooking. I would sit down and work out some alternatives such as lemon juice, ginger, curry powder or whatever. But when you are still getting salts from a lot of manufactured or processed foods your palate is not allowed to adjust downwards, it keeps being hiccoughed back up again which is why I think I still find salt the hardest.'

'I have no problems with money – I could go out and buy whatever I liked. The patients I work for are from the 'not particularly prosperous' parts of Yorkshire with a large number of Asians in the community and I am sure that the difference in the background of these people would produce totally different results.'

'We are vegetarians and we eat a lot of nuts. Steven in particular does as he has them for a snack, and we were trying to cut our fat intake so we had to cut down. Snacks – it is impossible to get something that is convenient, yet fits in with the recommendations. The second time I tried very hard to increase my carbohydrate but my meals are very bulky and it was very difficult and I felt permanently bloated for the second week.'

'I feel a disaster as a dietitian because I love ice cream and chocolate. I can eat as much as I want and do not put on any weight. My eating habits are quite ordinary – lunch is my main meal, which is at the hospital and none of the food at the hospital is high in fibre, they have baked potatoes but I do not like potato skins so the only fibre would have been those skins which I don't eat. All salad stuff is covered with mayonnaise or salad cream, or oil, so even if I take that it will be quite high in fat. By the end of the second week I tried to cut out sweets and ice cream but I went mad at the end of the study and ate more sweets in one day than I would normally eat, because I did not have my chocolate and I have cravings for chocolate and will eat a whole bar.'

'My parents are very traditional, old fashioned "meat and two veg" types – and they think we are pretty mad anyway as we are vegetarian. This was all too much. The other thing, apart from the social problem, was that they bring a food parcel, as they think we are so deprived; bags of crisps, cream cakes, and of course I ate them all. Because if they are there I will eat them.'

'I did not find it difficult at all.'

'My husband's only complaint was that his sodium intake was phenomenal without even including added salt and also he had a whole week on Shredded Wheat which is one of the salt-free cereals. His retort to that was that he does so much running and exercise that he felt he required his sodium so when the second one came round for him he decided he would not do it because he could not do it just for the sake of the sodium.'

'I was surprised how high my energy intake was. The recommended intake was 2150 and I was on 2732 without trying at all, but up to the time we received the results of our first survey we had been on 'gold top' milk for years. When the results came through, the second time round we went totally on to skimmed milk. It astonished me how much milk I was actually taking in tea as I drink mugs of tea as I like to take in a lot of fluid. The second time round, as well as going on to skimmed milk, I went off butter on to polyunsaturated fat and for the survey I just used polyunsaturated fat. I was interested to see that just by changing from 'gold top' to skimmed made a great difference in the proportions and I found that very useful to put over to patients that this is something that is not a great deal to alter in your dietary intake and yet is something that can make quite a dramatic difference.'

'I felt it was impossible for me to do it for more than four days.'

'It was difficult to sit at a hospital lunch next to people holding the salt cellar and pouring it liberally over their food. I was upset as I felt I was careful and I was amazed how much salt others in fact took when it was drawn to my attention.'

'We consumed a fair amount of milk in the family and I was quite surprised how easily we adapted from full-cream milk to skimmed milk, not being able to get semi-skimmed which I thought the kids would find easier to accept.'

'There is heart disease history in my family so I am very aware of all this. I get a kick out of eating healthy food and find an incentive in that, so this was no problem but I was a bit shocked to find that even on my good wicket I am not making the fat goal. I guess you have got to educate the food industry to put low-fat snacks out because it was the snacks that were knocking me I think. I take wholemeal sandwiches to work, so it is obviously the chipsticks, the biscuits and things like that, the snacks. You cannot keep eating huge meals.'

'From a professional dietetic point of view it was a useful exercise to remind us what we were putting on the plate, and what we were calling a portion of meat, or a slice of bread, and to check its weight. Sometimes in our mind's eye we overestimate when doing rough calculations with our patients. It was nice to be reassured on some and be reminded on others what portions and weights of separate foods look like. The hardest part was finding suitable, low-fat, low-salt fillings for the packed lunch. We happen to have a garden which is quite productive but if I had been paying for all those greengroceries I think I would have been rudely shocked.'

'As a non-dietitian, I was quite interested in taking part and very interested in the results as I really believed that our family dined correctly and ate the correct amount of food of different sorts. So, when I learned that our fat intake was too high I really was surprised and I cannot help believing that the general population's fat intake must be disastrously high. Cutting down on salt was no real hardship at all.'

'I was rather intrigued by the whole thing and did not mind doing it. We eat lots of wholemeal food, skimmed milk, not a lot of meat – so I thought it would be easy. When the figures came back I was very pleasantly surprised to see about the only thing which was wrong was the fat, which was too high. We had no problems with the fibre – we were floating in fibre! But when it came to fat that was the bogey one. Coming from the sort of background I do, where meat is eaten a lot of the time, and, knowing what my friends are like I don't think they've got a prayer of sticking to the guidelines at all.'

'I still eat crisps and chocolate but I think I will eat healthily when it is convenient. But I do feel healthy so I can't always be bothered now. I don't feel ill, I don't have a weight problem, and neither does my husband. If ever I feel really bloated I have a week or two where I am careful and then I lapse back. Even after the study I haven't changed as I have no real motivation. Healthy eating is only one part of a whole approach to life. Exercise, stress, smoking and drinking are also important.'

On further discussion it soon became apparent that one of the main 'problems' with eating in this way was that almost everyone consumed fewer calories. For some this was a positive joy and to most it was seen as an advantage for society as a whole given that so many people are overweight. But for the slim participants who lost weight they didn't need to lose it was something of a shock.

The answer to making up for the loss of calories which are condensed in fats and refined carbohydrate is to eat more food generally. If you can't keep up with the sheer bulk of food at one time then eat in between meals and let the body gradually adapt to more bulk at meals. This takes time to get used to and most of our participants simply did not have enough time to acclimatise themselves to the new pattern of eating required.

Question 2: Did you Find That you Lost Weight on This Diet?

'I normally eat quite a lot of high-energy snacks during the day and there is nothing readily available to hand that's high in energy yet still high in fibre and not fatty either, so I just tended to do without rather than eat a high-energy snack.'

'After the effort I was 11.5 per cent below my desired weight the second time. Basically I just could not consume any more bulk. But at weekends and in the evening I tried to push my intake up. But I just could not consume any more bulk at meal times.'

'We are all indoctrinated that potatoes, bread and cereals are not particularly good for you and I think there will be an incredible resistance there. I kept piling the spuds on my husband's plate and he thought he would get fat and gain weight but he didn't. He still has the equivalent of about three large potatoes on his plate in the evening and his weight in fact is still slightly dropping. He is reaping the benefit of the healthy eating of NACNE. I think the energy level goes down because fat and sugar takes up so much less volume than carbohydrate and you can't possibly make up all those calories with carbohydrate. I physically cannot eat it all at one meal and I do not have the time to eat it in between meals. It was suggested I should just drink more alcohol but I think that was not a good idea. I have got to eat a certain amount of fat or sugar, otherwise I will disappear. I am always hungry – it is a standing joke, and I feel I have to eat at least the minimum of what NACNE recommends otherwise it will be ridiculous.'

'We must warn underweight people that if they are cutting down the fat they will need a lot more carbohydrate.'

'My weight-loss was due to changing from gold top to skimmed milk and when it was very hot the milk went sour, so I changed to tea with lemon and the fact that I would normally have a lot of tea was relevant.'

'My calories dropped from 1800 to 1300 and I have maintained the ideas – I have only had one block of cheese since I did this. But I am finding it very difficult to replace the weight that I lost then, and there is always the temptation to have a Mars bar as I have lost the weight. I get pretty bored with sandwiches after the first three or four so I think it is going to be a problem for those who do not need to lose weight.'

Even though our participants tried very hard to adhere to the guidelines when they were at home, most found it difficult when eating out to come anywhere near the NACNE guidelines. As so many of them are working women who usually ate at least one meal a day out (in the hospital or other staff canteen) this was a real problem. Others found it almost impossible to eat out with friends and so simply turned down invitations to dine out during the study period for fear of doing serious 'damage' to their overall intakes for the week.

Question 3: What was it Like Eating Out at Work or for Pleasure?

'I feel that if you can generally stick to low-fat, low-sugar etc. then you can get away with it for a few meals and perhaps have a binge.'

'Eating out was a problem. I don't think it is impossible, it is just that you have to make food a different part of your life – to me it became more important and I was much more aware of it and I am not sure that I want to be that aware of it all the time. It would have to be a very important part of my life to achieve these goals, and I don't know that I want to be that food-conscious.'

'On the days when I have hospital food, or if I go out for a meal, no way am I anywhere near NACNE. Even if you go to a vegetarian restaurant, things are covered in fat. Eating out in say an Indian restaurant where so many of the dishes are vegetarian, many of the dishes are swimming in fat.'

'We gave up eating in the middle of the day in the hospital canteen a long time ago because the cheap meal was pizza and chips.'

'To meet the recommendations I would have to take a packed lunch and be prepared to cook every night at home and I am not prepared to do that when there is a meal available at work.'

'At work we had already introduced jacket potatoes about 6 months ago, wholemeal lasagne and wholemeal pastry on steak and kidney pies and things. But we have had to take the wholemeal pastry on steak and kidney pies off as the staff will not eat them. Some of it is the look of it – they do not look quite so crispy as the white.'

'We recently did a nutrition day where we cut out chips from the hospital menu and we were amazed how many took the jacket potatoes and wanted them. They had not seen them before and people loved them and are now asking for them. So, with a bit of pressure, the canteen aspect could be easily solved.'

Many of the participants found that they got hungry. They tried to overcome this by snacking between meals but soon realised just how difficult this was if it was not to wreck their overall plans for healthier eating.

Question 4: What About Snacks?

'We do not use a lot of convenience foods but there are always occasions when you feel you need them. It would be good if the manufacturers could aim to decrease the salt in convenience foods.'

'As well as better convenience foods, I think there are a lot of families who have lost the knack of cooking. Young mothers on the poverty line are out spending a lot of money on bad convenience foods and they need the education to go back to sensible cooking again as the knack of using fresh food is being lost.'

'I am at home all the time at the moment, my wife is the one who works, so it is easier for me to "snack" and since the second week I have been able to just go and peel a carrot, or have fruit, bread and jam, that kind of thing. So, at home it is easier but at work, surrounded by chocolate machines, it must be murder – I don't know how people manage. Where I was working I used to take my own lunch with my raw carrot, dried fruit etc. so that is one way of avoiding the pressures of the outside world, but it is hard work.'

'I cut out sweets and did not replace them with anything, digestive biscuits are not on sale at work, only chocolate machines. No banana machines! I think I got quite a lot of energy from sweets.'

'My boyfriend had to have sweets because he could not manage the bulk at meals and he was having snacks at mid-morning and mid-afternoon. We managed to fit in digestive biscuits as without meat and with cutting down drastically on the cheese we did have a fair amount of fat to spare. Digestives are quite good for calories and fibre.'

'We found nuts and raisins quite a good snack.'

'We liked malt loaf. I always wanted to put butter on it, but I did manage to eat it without. Actually I did not get through that much of it as I got a bit fed up.'

'It is also a matter of taste. I am not really fond of health food crunchy bars and I did have all the digestive biscuits handy and fresh fruit which I do enjoy eating, but I felt that I wasn't able to eat a snack because I was so full up from the previous meal. By forcing myself to eat more than I would normally to try and get the fibre intake up I felt I wasn't able to eat snacks the same.'

'I think I will go into business and make NACNE snacks – I am looking for a job. I'd be a millionaire if I could do it.'

Dietitians are obviously more aware of food types and groups than are most so we asked them to comment on the various food components when eating in this way.

Question 5: What are Your Thoughts About Various Individual Food Components When Eating Along These Lines?

Fat
'When speaking to patients about cutting down on their fat etc one of the biggest disadvantages is that they say, 'Oh you are cutting out all the good things in life', but I think if you are prepared to be a little more stringent with your day-to-day eating the odd meal out, bar of chocolate or home-made cake can be accomodated, if you obey the basic principles.'

'I am sure it is the meat that makes the most difference and that is why we keep our fat intake down and still drink whole milk and eat ordinary cheese.'

Protein

'People eat a lot of cheese, they can't afford lean meat, and it is good for sandwiches.'

'Having fresh meat available for sandwiches is a hassle for a lot of people, especially if you are trying to cut down on it and use fish or beans more. Then you haven't the fresh meat available for your sandwiches. Let alone the cost.'

Sugar

'I did wonder whether going back to having not quite steam roly-polys was more useful as then you are having sugar at meal times so you are restricting the sugar intake to three or four times a day rather than having lots of biscuits between meals which is the "kiss of death" as far as teeth are concerned. And yet the British people have been cutting down on puddings in a big way. To a certain extent they consume cakes and biscuits but not necessarily at a meal time.'

Fibre

'The biggest difficulty eating this way gets back to fibre again, I found getting my fibre up to about 30g a day was a big effort because I am such a small eater in the first place. I think it's worth inflicting this on the rest of the family in the long term but certainly not in the immediate short term because it would be very difficult to alter their eating patterns accordingly.'

'The government should make wholemeal bread cheaper than white, subsidise it or, like cigarettes, put a tax on white bread. Also they could intervene and help with the snacks.'

'I think that the price of standard wholemeal bread has got to be the same price as a standard white. At present the families who are short of money buy white sliced bread in the supermarkets as they can get more slices for their money. But I think the manufacturers of bread have got to adjust the price. When they are the same price you will have much less difficulty in convincing people.'

'If you want to increase your fibre you do not necessarily have to go overboard with the bran. I think you can get there by eating a certain amount of bread and wholemeal cereal as well as a normal helping of vegetables. We do not always have two veg and potato – people who come to our house always have potatoes with skins on whether they are boiled, jacketed or whatever. They turn up their eyebrows a bit the first time round but the second time they eat them.'

Question 6: Bearing in Mind That we Asked you to Make Pretty Major Changes Very Quickly, What Were the Difficulties?

'I just ate constantly in the day basically. The fibre fills you up very quickly and you find that you can't eat a great deal at once so within about an hour you are hungry again. I mostly ate fruit – I like fruit anyway and I eat a lot of fruit, but I certainly made friends with the fruit shop down the road from where I work.'

'I was hungrier and I was thinking much more about food.'

'It is grossly misrepresentational to have people having what you might call a standard British diet and then doing a massive change and trying to achieve the equivalent of 15 years in one week without having had the opportunity to think it through. That and coping with processed foods as they are at the moment and with other people's expectations when you eat out were great problems. This is why I feel that NACNE shouldn't be put down as an impossibility just because some dietitians couldn't do it. In fact, I don't *expect* dietitians to be able to do it because food is far more than just the working out of nutrients. It is what food means traditionally to you, your ritual in your life, the shopping and preparation of food, and that all needs to be thought through.'

'I felt permanently bloated and left every meal feeling that I had overeaten. With hindsight I would either introduce it over some months, or have more frequent meals, rather than keeping to my normal pattern of three extra-large meals.'

'If you are a vegetarian you are used to eating bulk but there is a limit to how much bulk even a vegetarian can eat at one sitting. I think this comes back to relying on things like NACNE snacks – if there are such things, between meals. I see this as the only way out of this dilemma.'

'Aside from fat, I think the expense was a major disadvantage. I found it much more expensive, mainly just trying to find something to replace cheese. It means going for lean meat and things which are expensive.'

'I found planning a menu the biggest disadvantage. It was harder work to consider everything, particularly when thinking of packed lunch fillings.'

'I think a convenience cook would not be able to afford the extra time taken.'

'I found it a bit of a disadvantage as we are a pudding family, especially fruity puddings rather than cheese and biscuits or just plain fruit – we have "afters". I found it very difficult and it would be impossible for me to eat like that all the time.'

'It was difficult fancying something and not being able freely to have a biscuit or something. I sensed a lack of freedom and I think I would have been happier not knowing about all the vitamins.'

'The major problem with much younger children is actually keeping their calories up as a low-fat diet is a very bulky diet and I don't think many little kids could cope with the bulk.'

Although almost all of our participants made great efforts for the duration of the study we felt that many would have found it difficult to keep up once the study was over. The next two questions addressed this problem.

Question 7: Could you Keep up Eating in This way for Ever?

'Yes, I think we could follow this way of eating. I might be a little worried about the children though. They are both under five at the moment and I would worry about the external pressures on them when they visit other houses. Certainly my wife and myself could follow it.'

'It has become a way of life for me.'

'I could go part-way, but not all the way; I could get my fat down. But I am feeding a husband who likes his fat too. I could probably meet the mid-way guidelines with a little imagination and a bit of time, and without so many salty processed foods.'

'Yes, I could live on this method, with the fat cut down. I cut down much more than I actually expected and I think I would relax that a bit as that was what I found difficult.'

'Yes, I can do it now because it is just me and if I got married I am sure I could do it but with older people such as my parents it would be a long struggle.'

'I think of the NACNE things there are some things people *could* adopt, the fibre one is obviously being adopted and is manageable, and I think a lot of people could *cut*, and have cut, for example salt intake and a lower sugar intake. I think it is the fat that is difficult for many people and certainly here in Yorkshire.'

'I would find it very difficult, particularly with two young children in the family, as I was concerned to change from whole milk to skimmed milk with the children. Also, it is very difficult to keep the children full without suitable snacks.'

'I could manage it but it would not necessarily be enjoyable until the day that low-fat, high-fibre snacks come along.'

'Yes, I think we could and I think the main reason is because we eat very little meat and fish, most of our fat intake is from cheese and I use very little in cooking.'

'I don't think it is for me as I could not meet the guidelines. I just happen to like all the wrong things. I know all the reasons why I should change my diet and I tell all my patients that they should change their diets, but it comes down to personal taste and I feel that NACNE goes too far.'

'Yes, and concerning the children, I can remember when I was young being constipated and having to have syrup of figs, even liquid paraffin. I cannot think that my children have ever been constipated.'

Opinions varied considerably from group to group. In one group of eleven only two thought it possible to keep up the good work whereas in another group of 10 in a different part of the country eight out of ten said they'd definitely keep it up.

Question 8: Have you in Fact Made any Permanent Changes as a Result of Doing the Study?

'Yes, what you will see in my cupboards and what is on my shopping list has changed, not quite to the extent of NACNE but that is just purely because I am not that organised. I was really good for a week, soaking my beans and being that one step ahead because I did really find that meat is a very convenient thing to cook. It cooks very quickly and if you are out at work and want a meal it is good. We do eat more pulses now, we still eat more fibre in the form of cereals and breads, and we eat a larger amount than we did of carbohydrate at our meals.'

'The diet gave me a chance to rediscover vegetables. For a long time I have just had cheese on toast for tea and a cooked meal at work, but not particularly any vegetables so it is nice to know they are not as bad as I remember them as a child. Doing it made me realise how easy it is to "get into a rut" with your food. It is easy to keep doing the same thing if you are in a routine, fairly busy and keep coming and going. It is good to have a change.'

'Well no, it couldn't become permanent. We have tried hard and I think we have cut out a lot of fat, we don't have as many sausages as we did. I used to be a "two-bags-of-crisps-a-day person" which I am beginning to modify, every now and again I have a day without a packet of crisps. We don't add as much salt as we used to. The biggest problem I think the general public would have is that whatever processed food you buy it has salt and sugar in it, even though you can't particularly taste the sugar. I think this is a big problem for the average person to go out and do their shopping.'

'My boyfriend was prepared to do it for a week, but not permanently. But then I suppose if it is supposed to be over 15 years, the changes must be gradual and presumably the food manufacturers are going to be changing if there is to be pressure from the public. The products will be available in the future. We wouldn't have too much trouble at all if processed foods were more healthy.'

'We now always have wholemeal crackers instead of water biscuits, which I love, but we have stuck to the wholemeal crackers, and we have crackers instead of bread. My husband is nagging me more now as he did enjoy the week when I put more effort in. I am getting positive encouragement from him so I am probably doing better than I would do on my own. We are not as good as we were but there have been permanent changes.'

'I have a husband who eats out and spends a lot of time at work eating food over which I have no control and I often comment that he does not eat properly, which I think is very common, especially with men. I was already not adding salt to vegetables, but I would always add the "pinch of salt" as I was taught to in baking, to bring out the flavour. Now I am not putting the salt into cakes etc. With the fat, I am trying to reduce the amount of sausages, beefburgers etc. and include more chicken, meat, stews, mince and take the fat off when I have cooked it, trying to be more conscientious and put a bit more effort in as it is so easy to rush tea because of piano lessons or whatever.'

'If making flapjack, for example, I will use half wholemeal and half white flour, and I try to include more wholemeal in all recipes.'

'I have stopped putting butter in my sandwiches, I now just have bread and a filling and we don't use salt in cooking or at the table any more.'

'I have changed to semi-skimmed milk from silver top and that goes down very well.'

'I am using more starchy foods now than I used to, many more wholemeal pastas and things and I am tending to do more vegetarian-type dishes with pasta and vegetables and not worrying about using meat any more. That is the biggest change I think I have made. In the supermarket I find myself continually looking into other people's baskets to see what they are buying that they shouldn't and I don't come out with as much any more. There are so many things I just don't want to buy any more. The labels have put me off. The whole thing has increased my personal awareness.'

When any professional group, and especially in the health-care world, lands on something it perceives to be of value it tends to become evangelistic, wanting to enforce its new-found views on others.

Dietitians spend a lot of their time trying to convince others to eat in ways that they otherwise might not so our next question sought to discover whether they felt that they should or indeed could impose the NACNE goals on others.

Question 9: Do you Think it is the Duty of a Dietitian to Influence her Family and Friends to eat More Healthily?

'I don't have a family, but I do try to influence my friends and have had some success; some have started to use wholemeal bread and low-fat spreads, but with others it is just a waste of time and I would not lose their friendship in trying to push them in the right direction.'

'I have inflicted it upon my children without telling them. I am quite surprised there was no hassle. The biggest hassle was not either of these weeks, but trying to change from butter. We did consume a considerable amount of butter and I felt very guilty. It was hard to find a suitable low-fat spread to suit everyone, at one time we had four kinds as everyone preferred something different!'

'I would not impose it on friends or family as I feel it is up to them to make the choice. We have children who have all left home but they visit at holiday time and we would encourage them to stick to that way of eating. We have grandparents who are in their 80s and no way will they take less salt in their food. They have lived to 85 with so much salt and they continue to pile it on and are not going to change now.'

'I thought it was interesting when Alan said he would not impose healthy eating upon visitors. I feel that if people are coming to eat with us they should eat what is going and I would feel it would be more of an imposition to fill them with sodium and cholesterol, rather than feed them relatively healthily. I think this ties in with dietitians feeling they should be slowly educating everybody.'

'I think making friends and family feel guilty when you visit them is more of a problem that the reverse.'

'Having heard I am a dietitian often people arrive with horror, but I do try to compensate in what I prepare; I try to make it reasonable, but then I say, "This is the special cream, this is our once-a-month cream and you are sharing it with us"; so we try to make a joke about it as well.'

'I feel that if my children go to a friend's house they must be able to eat there. If you set rigid rules and there is only white bread for tea they will say, "I am not eating that, my mummy does not give me that, that's poison etc." but to me it is not actually poison. It is not as good as wholemeal and I am just trying to keep it in moderation. Unfortunately, the moderation message has not got through!'

Almost all of us like to imagine that eating healthily paves the way for better health but there were other incentives our participants saw too.

Question 10: If you had to Encourage People to eat in This way What Incentives Would you Give Them?

'I think variety is one of the big benefits as all too often a lot of the patients we see consider meat and two veg and potatoes to be a meal and if you suggest things like brown rice or wholemeal pasta they say, "I couldn't get used to eating that", but they do.'

'With the percentage of the population who are overweight, the bulk and the "filling effect" of my diet must be one of the advantages while still being able to lose weight.'

'I don't find it a dull, monotonous diet, some people think vegetarian foods and pulses are monotonous but it does not have to be. But you must think about it. You can't just say instead of meat you will have pulses, you must make it into a main dish. But it is easy to do.'

'It was a revelation that the food tasted so good. The variety was really great. I really did enjoy food without salt.'

'I feel healthier for it. We went out about three weeks ago and I had a huge steak, dripping in fat, and at the end of it I felt ill – it was horrid. It was enough to make me turn vegetarian, I would not do it again. If you enjoy the food knowing that it is doing you good it gives you more incentive to eat healthy food.'

'With being in the "trade" I am aware that many things have additives and it gives me a nice feeling to think I am eating good, fresh, wholesome stuff, particularly the vegetables, as we grow them.'

'I can now look in the mirror and see my sylph-like figure and it is tremendous to think it is all because of the way I eat.'

In doing this Study the dietitians were both, so to speak, the hunters and the hunted so we asked them if, after trying to live along the lines of the goals set by us, they found the whole concept of goals or guidelines a workable idea at all.

Question 11: Is There any Sense at all in Having Dietary Goals or Guidelines Nationally?

'I think it is a good idea to have a goal but it depends what you mean by a goal. I certainly don't like the rigidity of something like the COMA Report with a particular percentage for an individual and I much prefer having a range for a group and I prefer talking about foods rather than nutrients. I prefer talking about eating more cereals, more bread, more fruit and vegetables and I think that is a much more sensible way of encouraging people to change their eating habits. It is certainly a much more practical way.'

'As a scientist, the essence of science is that you never know. There is no absolute, you have to say this is where we are right now, and on the basis of that we will come up with a hypothesis. I would suggest that with the NACNE study, but even more so with the COMA Report, a very well thought-out consensus has been reached and we can agree on it and I disagree with the view that we don't have enough information and that maybe because we are not *absolutely* sure we should not say anything.'

'Here is something we can at last hang our hats on and we ought to do it with conviction.'

'Yes, I think we need tight guidelines. I think the very experience of dietitians in this study is testimony to the fact that advice such as "eat more wholemeal bread, eat less fat" does not work if only because the dietitians themselves have been surprised they were not eating as healthily as they thought. They thought they were eating the right things and quantities but in actual fact a lot are not much better than Mrs Average anywhere.

I think overall I like to have a target and we have been discussing this today. We know that NACNE is there but to be realistic in Barnsley we are not going to get there in a very long time. Even so it is nice to have it at the end of the tunnel. I think the population likes figures, they love to know that they are on a 1000 calorie rather than simply a "reducing" diet and I think they prefer to do it that way as "moderation" methods have not worked. To say "cut down" or "increase" is not concrete enough. But I don't know whether NACNE has gone too far, it is a long-term thing and must be.'

'I think we must have something more concrete to work towards. We have mentioned the institutions, the hospitals, the school meals, we could talk about the prisons and all the other places which are responsible for people's welfare and I think where there is a nutritional adviser, or a dietetic adviser or an adequate catering adviser, there is no reason why, as we have done in our own homes, it should not be done in the institutions.'

'I do not particularly like goals at all. I think NACNE has gone too far and is unrealistic, both for myself and for my patients. I would find it very difficult to get any of my patients anywhere near NACNE here in Scotland. My people just would not follow that sort of diet. I think it would help if you had the food industry behind you, producing the sort of foods which you want and at a reasonable price. A lot of my people cannot afford wholemeal bread, it is as simple as that. It costs a few pennies more, but they still go on smoking, and they could probably afford it if they gave up smoking. Tinned fruit in natural juices is dearer than tinned fruit in syrup. Whatever you suggest is too dear and you have to be practical to them and you can't say, "This is what you've got to eat".'

'It is making people see what is going to benefit them and I think, (not talking about patients who are ill maybe with diabetes) that saying to somebody who is healthy now that they are going to live longer is beside the point. They are not bothered. You must show them some reason which is going to benefit them and this is very difficult and I don't know how to do it. You can tell them they are going to be healthy; that they are not going to have diseases; that they might live longer, and then they retort that they know somebody down the road who was on white bread all their life and they lived till 92!'

'People do not go shopping with health high on their food list – often the last thing they think about is the effect it has on their health. They eat it because they like it. But people who do change feel so much better and that is how I am trying to get people motivated by telling them the experiences of people who have changed. Up to two years ago, I never ate wholemeal bread, as I hated the stuff, I adored white bread and I ate it. I had been at college for three years, heard all the arguments and nothing anybody could say, lecturers or anybody, could make me want to stop eating white bread. But then I was medically advised to stop eating it – I had to start taking a high-fibre diet and I started taking wholemeal bread and hated it, but now I really do like wholemeal bread and do not eat white bread, and I do try to encourage my patients by telling them my story. And I stress that it does take a while to acquire the taste but I think a lot of people give up before acquiring the taste for it because if you do like white bread it is a very big change to wholemeal with a totally different taste.'

'I feel the goals are probably useful for us as health workers, but to the majority of our patients they would be totally useless. Even if you tried to explain them you would not make any impact, it would not make any difference to them. Most of my patients here in Leeds are Yorkshire people and I would be more than happy if they would reduce the amount of chips they have, and have Yorkshire pudding only three times a week instead of every day. In this area I feel we must get across basic changes first.'

'As professionals, I think it is time that, if we don't like what is being written, we must get out and write our own articles and saturate the press. And write it in great volume as what is read most often tends to linger longer in the mind. People become so aggressive when they read contradictory articles or see contradictory advertisements that in the end they are just confused and carry on the same way as before – neither is effective. This is why nationwide, dietitians must all say the same thing. Then everybody will have something to aim for.'

'I do think these goals are worthwhile. But there is no point in setting goals unless you expect people in some way to try to fulfil them. I don't think we as a nation are aware of what is a good, healthy diet and it is important to advertise it more openly and if that means setting national goals in some way it is perfectly acceptable. But then you have the problem that diet is about choice. With the variety of foods available inevitably people are going to make choices which are bad for them. So it is two-fold; you set national goals for individual people and then make them aware of them, but you cannot force them to achieve these goals.'

'I think the word dietary goal is good rather than fixed absolute guidelines because people's eating habits are generally entrenched for many, many reasons and dietary change, although it certainly does happen, is slow.'

'I think as far as sugar, fibre and salt are concerned, you could perhaps make out individual guidelines. For example, sugar – if your teeth are OK or if you have false teeth and you have no weight problem you could probably eat sugar. Salt – if you have not got a history of high blood pressure in the family and you are not overweight, perhaps you could tailor salt to fit your needs. Fibre – if your guts are working pretty well and you are quite happy with the way they are functioning and somebody sets a standard "the standard British stool" you could do that. But the one which is very difficult and calls for a blanket approach, as there is no way of testing individual risk, is fat. Maybe in the future science could tell us who are the people who need to watch out for it and who are most vulnerable.'

Perhaps the most potentially interesting thing about using dietitians to be their own 'victims' in this study was the impact that doing it could have on them as professionals whose job it is to give out information and instructions about food to others every day. For most, doing the study taught them something in this sphere and for some it was a chastening experience. Our last question sought to find out how they thought the study had altered their performance as professionals.

Question 12: How has Taking Part in This Study Altered the way you Work or Think as a Professional Dietitian?

'It was important for me to see that it could be done. I am not less tolerant of patients as a result but I can give them real advice about what to do. It helped me with practical advice. Changing eating habits is one of the most difficult things we can ask people to do.'

'The whole of my working life has been concerned with nutrition education and I felt in order to be able to do it successfully I had to see if I could do it myself as well as giving practical examples. Also, I have had two children in that time and I am now much more tolerant. Food habits are very difficult to change as it is so much more than nutrition. I have got much more realistic about my aims. And perhaps I will work harder at things which are achievable.'

'With dietetics you have got to achieve modifications which are realistic. With your 70-year-old diabetic it is no use saying "eat wholemeal bread" if they are used to white bread. You can only say that it is a good idea if you cut the sugar out of your tea and don't have puddings too often.'

'I think I am a lot more positive now that I have done it myself. I hope it has enabled me to say, "Look I have tried it, I've tried it this way, I've tried it another way, why don't you try it a different way?" I don't give up easily with people, I am very tolerant. But having done it I perhaps can be more forceful in the advice that I offer and say, "Look, it *is* possible", and then try to explore other things with them. Also, it has changed my relationship with other people. Perhaps I am more convinced that I should go out and preach more than I did. Also I have had a go at one or two supermarkets recently as I got so frustrated when I was shopping – they had run out of wholemeal crackers or something.'

'Having done it you can picture physically what a NACNE meal does look like and say to people, "Look you did not need those chips, eat a jacket potato instead". Weighing things increased my ideas of portions. I do get frustrated in supermarkets now and don't want to buy the junk. Why should I? But I see others buying it and I just want to tell them. Patients say to you, "Should I eat wholemeal bread?" Before I used to say to them, "You should", and *now* I say "*yes*, you really *ought* to".'

'I think it is dangerous to be too evangelical about this, you might get a back-lash effect with people. They think they have heard all about dieting before.'

'We have an obesity clinic and all our patients are meant to be on a high-fibre diet, but if a patient turns to me and says they hate wholemeal bread, I do not tell them they must have it or they can't be on the diet. I would tell them to take white bread and count their energy portions, but I do try to encourage them to take the high-fibre diet. I tell them it is an acquired taste so try it and see if they can get used to it. But I do not see any point in telling them they must eat high-fibre as I know they will go home and they won't.'

'I have become interested in reaching a wider range of people. Before, I felt my priorities were with people who were referred for therapeutic diets. I have become more interested in reaching more of the population, people who don't necessarily need a therapeutic diet, but just need educating. That is my biggest change – my interest in that area.'

'No, I don't think I have altered the advice I give but I am probably more sympathetic to my patients' failings. I don't think it has altered the actual nature of the advice that I have given but it has made me a bit more practical about what portions are and you began to know what ounces and grams looked like.'

'I think I was quite sceptical as to how we could implement NACNE when it first came out. I held my hands up in horror and did not think we could do it all at once. The survey has shown me that we can't do it all at once, but it has made me more positive in trying to help people by offering the information in a different way and perhaps by homing-in on what they *can* achieve, and what is going to be beneficial now to them, in the hope of building on it in the future. And on the practical aspects such as asking patients to do weekly records etc. I am far more sympathetic towards them now.'

'I feel I have a better understanding and the salt is the main thing I am stricter about. Also I am more specific about quantities.'

'Certainly I can relate much better in a practical sense to telling them how to achieve meals and menus with less salt and less fat.'

'I think in general it will have helped the dietetic profession to realise the practical problems and make them much better able to advise their clients or large groups. I also think that it will have helped us personally as dietitians and I am very pleased that the BDA set this up.'

The contents of this chapter can only scratch the surface of all the valuable information and practical tips that came out of both the study itself and the interviews. Because of this and because the whole idea of the study was to produce practical, workable, guidelines for healthy eating based on NACNE, we gathered together all the valuable tips from our participants and have made them into a whole chapter of their own. The next chapter summarises what we have learned.

CHAPTER FIVE

What Have we Learned?

Introduction

Quite obviously none of us enjoys being ill or watching other members of our family suffer from heart disease, cancer or diabetes, or indeed any illness we know *could* have been prevented. Today we can make at least some strides towards better health by eating more wisely. However, having said this, when we think about food, probably the first thing we think of is that we want to enjoy it. But how *can* we enjoy it if we are made to feel guilty that we are not eating the right foods, or if we are worrying about how much we are paying for our food, or find that it takes too long to prepare? As we saw in the Introduction, food fulfils so many roles in our lives that to simply look at it as a source of nutrition is to miss the point.

The suggestions in this chapter are to help you enjoy your food, in the knowledge that it is leading you or your family to better health at the same time. Healthy eating does not have to be boring or 'goody-goody' – it can be tasty, full of variety and even fun!

Before starting to think about the sort of food we should be choosing, let's not lose sight of the fact that the desire to eat is a natural instinct. Without food none of us would survive. However, food is not only used for physically maintaining and repairing our bodies, but also as a reward – as a way of coping with life. Although this book is no place for discussing all the psychological aspects of eating, we cannot ignore the fact that unhappy relationships, the lack of stable relationships or indeed any dissatisfaction with life can influence people's dependency on food as a reward. This is especially true for women, who have fewer culturally-acceptable reward systems than men. For many women, bringing up children and running a home are undervalued, and they therefore suffer almost permanently from low self-esteem and consequently feel the need to reward themselves in other ways. Some blow a lot of money on clothes, some have affairs, some drink and others eat. Men more easily obtain reward from achievement at their work, through their hobbies and clubs and, unlike women, the reward of food is less readily available to them during their working day.

In this chapter we look at all the lessons that have come out of the study and see how they can be applied to all of us in our day-to-day lives.

Unfortunately, many people equate healthy eating with boring, unattractive eating – which is a mistake.

In no way is a healthy approach to eating intended to spoil your enjoyment when eating, or to increase the guilt associated with eating (a feeling commonly linked to eating by women). Most people have lost patience with comments such as 'you have no willpower if you eat that!'; or 'you shouldn't be giving that food to your husband, wife or children'.

Let's start off by getting a few things straight. There is no such thing as bad food and good food; most food is nutritious, at least to some degree. It is more a question of which foods should be best eaten on a regular, day-to-day basis and which are best used only occasionally.

Two important obstacles to eating healthily are *time* and *money*. Healthy products, for example reduced-sugar preserves, reduced-fat cheeses, wholewheat or high-fibre pasta, wholemeal bread, canned fruits in natural juice and products free of preservatives and additives, all tend to cost more than their less healthy equivalents. In addition, hunting out these products takes more time when shopping and may involve travelling further and even to several different shops. It is also true that producing enjoyable meals that conform to our healthy eating model, and to do so without using convenience foods, can take a lot more time.

Other obstacles to healthy eating include:

- poor availability of healthy meals and foods, particularly in small grocers, supermarkets, cafés, restaurants, canteens and from take-aways (see page 182)
- catering for the individual tastes of a whole family, particularly with young children and when entertaining
- knowing what to choose to eat.

So obviously it is not that easy – you can only do your best! It is by continually and slowly adopting new healthy eating habits that change occurs which then becomes a habit. No one can reasonably expect us, when shopping, to spend more than a few pence extra a week, or to take more than a few minutes extra in our attempts to eat healthily. Nor could we be expected to spend more than a few minutes extra when cooking or tracking down a better restaurant, café or take-away – not unless we have plenty of time to spend. As the demand for healthier products increases life for the discerning eater will become easier; the volume of sales will go up, the costs will come down and more suitable convenience foods will become available. The secret is to keep showing that there is a demand!

All this is worthwhile because healthy eating makes life more enjoyable because it makes us feel fitter and helps us keep free from the diseases of the affluent Western world which are mainly food-based.

Ideas on what foods and habits to adopt for a healthier way of eating and how to overcome some of the obstacles are discussed on the following pages. Suggestions are made, for example, for cost savings on foods which can be balanced against the higher cost of the healthier variants of manufactured foods.

What to Aim For

The goals set for the participants in the Study related to fibre and complex carbohydrate, fat (both its amount and type), sugar, salt and alcohol. Each of these will be looked at separately. It should be appreciated that it is a healthy diet *overall* that is important. If you lead a busy life, eat to a budget and depend on convenience foods you cannot expect to hit every goal *every* day. You may find a wholemeal pizza, wholemeal quiche or wholemeal malt loaf in the shops; buying these will help to increase your fibre intake. But to control your fat, salt and sugar consumption as well, you would need to eat home-made versions with carefully chosen ingredients. However, on other days you may balance things out by eating white bread with a low-fat cheese, or a low-salt spreading fat and a reduced-sugar jam.

Trying to limit your foods to just those which really meet all the criteria, in terms of fats, fibre etc. is fine if you can cook a variety of foods yourself. If time is against you and manufactured food is a necessity then limiting your diet in this way could become very monotonous. In fact, narrowing your diet to just a few foods could in fact lead to a deficiency in vitamins, minerals, essential amino acids (which come from proteins) or essential fatty acids. This is the difference between eating healthily and becoming a 'health food nut'. It may be helpful at this stage to look back to Chapter 3. As was mentioned there, (pages 38 to 56), some of the achievers did buy sausages, cream, crisps or chocolate biscuits, but they were in the minority. One can safely say that the study's healthy eating goals can be achieved by occasionally buying sausages, pâté, crisps, cream, cakes, pastry, preserves, sauces and pickles. However should they all appear on the shopping list each week then the healthy way of eating would be difficult to achieve.

The diagram on pages 48 to 49 may also act as a guide of what to aim for. This shows some of the differences between the diet of the YES group and that of the NO group and hence the sort of beneficial changes expected of the UK population. There are however two qualifying points. Firstly, the NO group already had a diet nearer the goals than the average person, so the difference is less than the change required by the nation as a whole. Secondly, improving one's diet does not mean making overnight changes. Therefore the sort of differences between the YES and NO groups represent ample change for most people to aim for in the next year or so.

Children in the Household

Many of the participants in the Study who had young children commented that this greatly influenced their choice of foods.

Looking around the world it is apparent that children from different cultures eat quite different food, but that the food is very similar to their own family's diet. The likes and dislikes of young children are to a large degree based on what is familiar to them. Children who are introduced first to wholemeal bread may well later reject white bread and vice versa. Similarly, children brought up in vegetarian families will quite happily eat bean and nut dishes and will find meat distasteful or unpalatable. So it is quite possible for families with young children to adopt healthy eating principles as a way of life – it is more a question of what they are used to. Obviously, changes are difficult at any age but children, with their desire to be like others they know, are often more resistant to change than are adults. Many parents, not wanting to make their children appear 'odd' to their friends and because they don't want to take the risk of losing their children's love by 'forcing' them to eat things they don't really like, buckle under the pressures and give in to eating habits they know are not in their children's best interests. The truth is that we are not depriving our children of love by refusing to give them junk foods – though we *are* depriving them of illness and suffering later in life, because they will grow up to be healthier.

Unfortunately, the problems of enforcing healthy eating *today* are very real but the dangers of ill health forty years from now are very *unreal* to most of us. This makes us favour the short-term gain more often than not.

But children are amazingly flexible and can take change very well, even from a very early age. We found that in some of our families the children really helped lead the way to healthier eating.

The following reactions from young children are not uncommon: two boys, five and seven years old, staying with relatives said 'We don't want that white bread, we want that super bread, with little grains on it' (the wholemeal bread!). A three- and a five-year-old, spotting a nut roast to be eaten after they had gone to bed said 'You will let us have some tomorrow, won't you?' The four-year-old son of a mother trying to eat according to our goals said, 'Too much fat isn't good for you'; he also asked his mother for fewer biscuits!

Some Do's and Don'ts with Young Children

- Try where possible to introduce children to a healthy way of eating right from the start. Go straight from breast feeding to wholesome, unrefined foods. As the child grows up let chips and high-fat, high-salt foods such as burgers and sausages be the exception rather than the rule.
- Introduce food changes to the family slowly. Sudden changes are likely to cause difficulties. For example, you are unlikely to succeed in trying to replace sausages, burgers, chips and white bread overnight with more bean dishes, wholemeal rice, wholemeal bread and jacket potatoes. Go for one change at a time and when you have made a significant impact with this, go for another goal. Some gradual changes include adding beans to favourite meals, or introducing wholemeal bread by preparing sandwiches with one side white and one side brown.
- Offer new foods you are trying to introduce to children in fun shapes and small finger-sized pieces.
- The fibre content of children's diets should not be suddenly increased as this could lead to several motions being passed daily. They will find this odd or even worrying so go slowly.
- Similarly, the sugar and fat content of children's diets should not be decreased too rapidly. For normal-weight children, quite a lot of extra cereals and starchy vegetables need to be eaten to keep up the calories they need. It takes time to adjust to the sheer bulk of food that needs to be eaten to achieve this. Children given 'whole foods' from weaning age fare perfectly well and children brought up in this way will never have had added salt or sugar and do not need it.
- Make healthy eating fun. It should not be a chore inflicted on children. Rules such as 'don't eat sweets, crisps and sausage rolls when you go to your friend's party' probably

do little to improve health. Furthermore, such rules probably go a long way towards creating complexes about food and create family tension. When other people's children come to your house you can offer them a healthier choice of snack foods. You will be amazed how many of these go down a treat and how great an influence this can be on that child's family's eating when it returns home talking about the lovely food at your house. Some suggestions are included in the section on entertaining.

Children are very much creatures of habit – they like what they are used to. Many mothers of families who eat sensibly say 'It's funny, my children nearly always choose the fruit and vegetables, they are not really bothered about sweets.'

• Normal toddlers will refuse food some days, eat large amounts other days and have crazes on certain foods, whilst rejecting others. This is all part of growing and developing. Approached in the right way, this behaviour should not disrupt the adoption of healthy eating practices in your family.

Keep mainly wholesome foods in the house, so that food craving is answered by developing a taste for basic foods with good nutritional value, such as breakfast cereal, toast, fruit, cheese etc, rather than sweets, biscuits or crisps. To some extent you can go along with food crazes during toddlerhood. The toddler's body may know better than you what it needs. Don't get up-tight when he or she refuses food. Your child is probably not hungry. Don't offer tempting foods of poor nutritional value as an alternative. This will just set up a game in which children manipulate you – a game which you are almost bound to lose because you dare not run the risk of putting your love on the line in the 'food-shows-them-that-you-love-them' battle.

Perhaps the safest line of thinking with young children is that if you haven't got it in the house they can't eat it and that if they are really hungry they will eat something else instead. If the 'something else' is wholesome, colourful and comes with your approval it will soon become acceptable. One last thing, don't tell children they should be eating things 'for their own good' or for the good of their health'. They see other children who seem perfectly healthy to them and yet they eat 'junk' food and long-term threats of future ill-health simply don't have any impact. To a child under 16 anyone over 20 is old and over 40 ancient, so it is hardly surprising they get ill is it?

As with most things with children, example is the best teacher. Your kids will do what you do when it comes to eating and this works for good and evil.

But feeding your family well pre-supposes that you have got the right sorts of food available at home to give them and the starting point for this is shopping.

Shopping for Health

There are lots of important factors that influence where you shop, such as time, transport, where you live, value for money, the shop's environment, habit, familiar faces, or lack of crowds and pressure.

There are also many reasons why you choose particular foods. These include:

cost
your own taste
habit
how hungry you are
the tastes and preferences of others
whether you want to treat or comfort yourself, or someone else (and this might be a perfectly unconscious motive)
the occasion
the look of the food
special offers
the packaging
the shopping and cooking time you have available
what you think the food will do for your health
the food labels
advertising
wanting to make an impression when entertaining
a way of expressing your love or care for others.

Making changes in the way you eat may mean altering your shopping practices. You therefore need to think why you shop where you do and why you choose particular foods. You will probably find that some things you do are essential to your lifestyle, whilst others are less so.

The dietitians and their friends and relatives who undertook our study found time an important factor when trying to eat more healthily. Generally, most of the participants did not change where they shopped, nor did they find shopping more difficult than usual. However, we should not forget that a few did find their shopping was more difficult and this has to be balanced against hardly anyone finding the shopping easier. It is also fair to mention that many of our participants were already shopping where a variety of whole foods were available.

You may have already found the best places to shop for your way of life, in which case simply making a few changes in what you choose to buy may be appropriate for you. However, there are suggestions on where to find healthier foods in each of the sections on fibre (page 102), sugar (page 117), fat (page 131) and salt (page 146). There are also suggestions in the section on balancing the cost on where to shop to make cost savings (page 175). But here are some general hints on shopping:

- The larger the supermarket, the more likely you are to find a range of healthy products.
- When you can, shop at non-peak times so that it is easier to look for different products and to ask for help from the shop's staff.
- Always check the date stamping on products when you are unfamiliar with them to avoid any food wastage.
- The mark-up on some healthy variations of common food products is not necessarily any greater in a small supermarket compared to a large one (although generally most products are cheaper in the larger stores or large supermarket chains).
- You can make many changes to your diet without shopping in new shops – by the time you are ready for further changes, other 'improved' products may well have reached

your usual shops. An interesting thing here is that if you and your friends really want a supermarket to stock a particular item just keep telling the manager about it – not all together but individually. Experience shows that this gentle pressure works: after all, he is in business to stock what people want to buy. For more on this, see below.

- Try to write a shopping list if you are making a few changes to your shopping pattern – although it is always a good habit anyway. When writing the list, think about the number of meals you are shopping for; how long the foods will last in the storage that you have available; and what is in season. This will save wastage or running short of food.
- It is not a good idea to go shopping when you are hungry, angry, anxious or feeling over-full, as these will all distort your food selection.
- Learn to read and understand the food labels.
- Never be afraid of asking the shop's staff for help.

Asking for Help when Shopping

When you cannot find the healthy food you are looking for, do ask the shop assistant. There may be fewer numbers of packs of the healthy lines, making them more difficult to spot. They may have sold out, in which case you will be letting the shop know the demand exceeds their stocks. This sort of approach comes quite naturally to some shoppers and should be much more common than it is. As a nation we British tend to be too reserved and polite about what is available and forget that the shop is there to serve *us* and cater for our needs.

Taking this one stage further by exerting more pressure for healthier food comes easier to some people than others. For example, some people may feel able to ask to see the manager of the store and discuss:

- why they do not stock more of a particular healthy line *or*
- whether they could stock a healthy line you have seen elsewhere *or*
- the selling of an easily-imagined food item that you have never seen before such as a lower-sugar biscuit, or a biscuit made with polyunsaturated fat, *or*

- you could discuss the siting of the healthy foods if they have been difficult to find and mention their cost compared with the similar 'standard' product.

Comments like these do bring results. You may also like to suggest that these matters are discussed with the shop's head office, or you could even write to the head office yourself if you feel sufficiently motivated.

Thankfully there is a growing trend to sell healthy products alongside traditional products (for example, wholemeal bread next to white bread). This is a step in the right direction. Putting healthy foods in a special 'health food' section encourages us to feel different or even 'freaky' and can create suspicions in certain people. If such foods are sorted away in a special area they can be difficult to find and will almost certainly discourage newcomers from trying healthier products which will in turn tend to maintain the current price differential between these and other foods. Given that impulse buying is so important, healthy foods must be as easily available, well packaged and advantageously priced as 'normal' foods if nutrition education is to have its maximum effect.

Storing Food

An important part of enjoying a healthy diet is storing food properly. Poor storage can lead to waste and increased food costs, to eating deteriorated food with a poor flavour or at worst to eating unfit and thus unhealthy food.

Apart from noticing any date marks, it is important to take notice of storage conditions recommended by food manufacturers. The date marks are based on the assumption that the food will be properly stored.

Some Basic Information About Food Labelling

One of the greatest problems our participants found was that it was difficult or even impossible to know what foods actually contained. This makes healthy eating a difficult business and changes are afoot to improve matters. As things stand at the moment all pre-packed foods and most non-pre-packed foods must show the name of the food on the label. Some names are *prescribed* by law such as wholemeal bread. Other foods have *customary* names such as 'pizza' or 'muesli'. Foods that have neither customary nor prescribed names have a descriptive name, for example 'crunchy peanut butter' or 'thyme, parsley and lemon stuffing mix'. These names need to be precise enough to distinguish them from other similar products. The proper name of the food can then be used in conjunction with a brand name or trade mark. The form the food is in should be stated unless it is absolutely obvious, for example dried, smoked, ready-mixed and so on.

Misleading names are not permitted, for example, 'vanilla essence' means that the flavour comes from the vanilla pod; 'vanilla flavouring' means the flavour is largely simulated. Similarly, yoghurts named 'strawberry' or 'strawberry flavoured', or yoghurt cartons with pictures of strawberries on them must have their flavour coming mainly from real strawberries. The words 'strawberry flavour' means the flavour comes mainly from artificial flavourings.

Most pre-packed foods must include a complete list of INGREDIENTS – current exemptions include fresh fruit and vegetables which have not been peeled or cut into pieces; vinegar made from a single product; flavourings; cheese, butter, fermented milk and fermented cream which contain only lactic products, enzymes, micro-organism cultures and salt (in the case of cheese), which are essential to their manufacture. Curd cheese is an exception. There are some other foods which are exempt generally from food labelling. These include cocoa and chocolate products; honey; milk and certain condensed and dried milk products; hen's eggs; coffee and coffee products; food prepared on domestic or similar premises for charitable sales; and foods in very small packages.

The ingredients on labels are shown in descending order of weight. Added water must be shown if it makes up more than 5 per cent of the finished weight.

Food ADDITIVES are included on the list of ingredients. These additives are used for colouring, flavouring, sweetening and for preserving or enhancing keeping qualities or to affect the texture or consistency of foods (emulsifiers, stabilisers, thickeners and gelling agents). Other additives include foaming agents, flour improvers, glazing agents and raising agents. Only additives which are currently considered safe and necessary are permitted by law. The use of additives is controlled by the Minister of Agriculture, Fisheries and Food, together with the Secretary of State for Social Services.

Most additives are given an E number agreed by the member states of the European Community. For example:

colours are in the E100 series
preservatives are in the E200 series
antioxidants are in the E300 series
emulsifiers, stabilisers, thickeners or gelling agents in the E400 series.

Most foods have to carry a DATE MARK if their minimum durability is less than eighteen months. Exceptions include fresh fruit and vegetables which have not been peeled or cut into pieces; flour; confectionery (such as cakes and buns) and bread (which are normally eaten within 24 hours of being made); vinegar; cooking salt; solid sugar and products made mainly from flavoured or coloured sugars; chewing gum; deep frozen foods; ices; and cheeses intended to ripen in the packaging.

Other foods with a life greater than three months must have a date mark indicating the end of the month and year by which they should be eaten. Food with less than a three-month life must show the day and the month by which they should be eaten. In this case the year is not required. When a label has a 'sell by' date rather than a 'best before' date, then the label should also tell you within how many days of purchase the food should be eaten. At the time of writing, new labelling laws particularly relating to fat content are being drafted.

What to do if you Have a Complaint About a Food or its Labelling

First, try your shop or the manufacturer. If this does not deal with your problem you can go to your local authority who are responsible for enforcing the law on food labelling. In England and Wales (except London) go to your Trading Standards Officer at your county council. In some cases you may be referred to your local Environmental Health Officers. In London and Scotland you need to go directly to your Environmental Health Officers. In London they work for the borough councils and in Scotland the district councils. In Northern Ireland the Public Health Inspectors of the district councils are the people to approach. To keep up to date on food labelling and to know what the E numbers stand for, write to the Ministry of Agriculture, Fisheries and Food or buy a reliable book on the subject.

In England and Wales information is available from:

Ministry of Agriculture, Fisheries and Food
Lion House
Willowburn Trading Estate
Alnwick
Northumberland NE66 2PF

In Scotland from:

Scottish Home and Health Department
Foods Branch
Room 40
St Andrew's House
Edinburgh EH1 3DE

In Northern Ireland from:

Department of Health and Social Services
Medicines and Food Control Branch
Annexe A
Dundonald House
Upper Newtownards Road
Belfast BT4 3SF

As we saw in the chapter about the NACNE Report it did not concern itself with everything to do with healthier eating – it looked mainly at the changes that could and should be made to the main foodstuffs we eat.

Because there are still so many misconceptions about even

these common foods we thought it would make sense here to outline the facts as they are currently perceived. Let's start by looking at dietary fibre or roughage.

Taking the Rough with the Smooth: Eating More Fibre and Starchy Foods

What is Fibre?

Dietary fibre is the name given to a whole range of complex plant substances which pass right through the intestine and bowel without being absorbed. It not only aids digestion, but also helps prevent constipation.

What do we Mean by Starchy Foods?

These are the cereals and starchy vegetables which, when eaten in a whole or unrefined form, are present with their dietary fibre. They need to be cooked before eating.

How to Eat more Fibre and Starchy Foods

- Eat more foods which come from plants e.g. bread, flour, breakfast cereals, oats, rice, fruit, potatoes, beans and other vegetables.
- Choose high-fibre foods in preference to the lower-fibre ones.
- High-fibre foods absorb more water in your body so you'll need to drink more fluid.

High-fibre choice	Low-fibre choice
Wholegrain wheat and bran breakfast cereals*	Sugar-coated cereals* Rice breakfast cereals
Wholewheat, rye, mixed wholegrain, granary, and brown breads.* Wholewheat and wholegrain are best	White bread
Wholewheat and brown flour	White flour
Wholemeal pasta, brown rice, whole oats, maize, barley	Ordinary pasta White polished rice
Pulses e.g. baked beans*, kidney beans, soya beans, lentils, chick peas etc, nuts, seeds	Cheese*, eggs, fish*, meat*
Fresh and dried fruit and nuts	Sweets
Wholemeal, oat and bran biscuits* Wholemeal, rye or bran crispbreads*	Other biscuits* – sweet and savoury
Jacket potatoes, other vegetables and salads	

*may be high in salt – read the label.

What are the Main Sources of Fibre in our Diet?

48 per cent comes from vegetables
30 per cent from cereals and bread
10 per cent from fruit
12 per cent from nuts and seeds

What Sort of Differences are There Between High and Low-fibre Choices?

High-fibre choice	% fibre	Low-fibre choice	% fibre
Wholemeal bread	8.5	White bread	3
Wholemeal flour	9.5	White flour	3
Weetabix	13	Rice Krispies	4.5
Wholewheat pasta (raw)	10	White pasta (raw)	3
Wholegrain rice (raw)	5	White rice (raw)	2
Potato in its jacket	2.5	Boiled potato	1
Lentils (raw)	12	Beefburger	0
Kidney beans (raw)	25	Mince	0
Orange	2	Orange juice	trace
Banana	3.5	Boiled sweets	0

You may see different figures quoted elsewhere, this is because different analytical methods give slightly higher or lower values.

What About Bran?

Eating unprocessed bran – the outer coating of cereals (usually sold as wheatbran) – can help to prevent and cure constipation. However, this is not really the answer to improving your diet. It is not just fibre you need increased, but starchy foods as well. It is therefore more fibre-rich, carbohydrate foods in general that you need to eat. One of the reasons you should eat 'whole' or unrefined foods is to make sure your body receives all the vitamins and minerals that are otherwise removed in the processing of white cereals (such as white flour and white rice). In cereals there is a concentration of vitamins and minerals in the germ. When white flour is milled, most of the germ and bran are removed, so if you eat white flours and breads and add bran back into your diet, you are still losing out on all the goodness contained in the germ.

In fact it might be possible to do yourself harm by taking too much added bran. It has been suggested that bran can interfere with the absorption of some minerals, leaving a shortage in the body. As the high-fibre, unrefined foods are themselves richer in vitamins and minerals, they are unlikely to cause such a deficiency.

On the whole look out for wholegrain foods rather than foods with added bran, in other words, eat your bran where it naturally belongs, in the unrefined food along with a good supply of vitamins and minerals.

Shopping for Fibre and Starchy Carbohydrate

Thankfully high-fibre foods are becoming more widely available in the shops. The following can all be found in most *large supermarkets*:

Wholewheat pasta e.g. spaghetti, spirals, macaroni or lasagne (and high-fibre white pasta)
Wholegrain (brown) rice
Wholemeal bread in large and small loaves, rolls and baps
Wholemeal muffins
Wholemeal pitta bread (an assistant manager in one of Sainsbury's largest stores said 'the wholemeal pitta sells better than the white, but this is not true of scones')
Wholemeal fruit buns and loaves, or muesli buns or wholemeal malt loaf
Rye breads and mixed grain breads (high-bran breads)
Wholewheat spaghetti in tomato sauce
Wholewheat flour – often only a strong bread-making variety but sometimes self-raising
Oat cakes
Baked beans, canned kidney and butter beans and sometimes other canned beans in brine or sauce
Dried beans, lentils and split peas – rarely a wide choice
Wholegrain breakfast cereals, e.g. Puffed Wheat, Shredded Wheat, Weetabix, wheatflakes, unsweetened muesli, (bran breakfast cereals e.g. All Bran, Branflakes)
Wholemeal pizzas and flans
Ready-made wholewheat lasagne, ravioli, cannelloni etc
Wholemeal scone and crumble mixes
Fresh fruits and vegetables

Frozen and canned fruits and vegetables, although the skins are often removed, e.g. tinned pears and peaches, or tinned potatoes

Dried fruits – choose carefully because these are often plumped up with mineral oil and sometimes coated with sugar or glucose syrup

Nuts, e.g. unsalted peanuts, almonds, walnuts, hazelnuts and sometimes brazil and cashew (but remember that most nuts have a high fat content)

For those shopping in smaller supermarkets or grocer's shops, it might not be so easy as some of these foods will probably not be stocked. To have a wide variety of high-fibre foods you may need to stock up following a visit to a larger supermarket or hypermarket, or track down a health food or wholefood shop to supplement your local supermarket's produce.

In addition to the more basic high-fibre foods found in your supermarket, high-fibre foods most easily found in your *health or wholefood shop* include:

Wholegrain pudding rice

Fine wholewheat flours and self-raising wholewheat flour

Other wholegrain flours, e.g. buckwheat, maize, rice, rye and soya

Brown semolina

Jumbo oats

Rolled and wholegrain barley, rye, wheat and millet

Bulgar and cracked wheat grains

Peanut butter without additives

A wide variety of pulses, i.e. beans, lentils etc

A wide variety of nuts, e.g. cashew, tiger as well as basic peanuts, almonds etc

Sunflower, sesame and pumpkin seeds

Dried fruit without additives

Unsweetened muesli – often a choice

A range of wholewheat pasta, e.g. rings, spirals, lasagne, shells etc.

Complete pasta dishes, e.g. ravioli, cannelloni etc

Wholemeal stuffing mixture

Reading the Labels

Try to read the labels and check that you are buying wholegrain, wholewheat or wholemeal. Where possible choose these rather than a white product with bran added (which still has some of the valuable vitamins and minerals removed).

Where products say 'brown' this means that they have more fibre than the 'white' product but that some of the fibre has been removed. Also be warned that there are products which have *some* wholemeal or wholegrain cereal but that the rest of the product is just wheatflour or another refined flour. The term 'wheatflour' means that the flour comes from wheat but it may be white. Remember to look out for the sugar, fat and salt on the label. Some wholegrain products can be very high in fat, such as wholemeal pork pie, or in sugar, like a wholemeal malt loaf.

What About Price?

As a general rule the shop with the fastest turnover is likely to be the cheapest. Sometimes buying food loose or in bulk in a wholefood shop can reduce the price.

Nuts tend to be a little cheaper in health food or wholefood shops and so sometimes are pulses, mueslis and flours, especially when bought loose or in bulk. Where a high-fibre product is well 'hidden' in the supermarket – behind a pillar or at the back of a top or bottom shelf, it might be found cheaper elsewhere.

A study of prices in a large supermarket (in February 1985) found the following price differentials between the refined and unrefined high-fibre products:

- wholemeal spaghetti – 37 per cent more than white spaghetti
- wholemeal macaroni – 33 per cent more than white macaroni
- brown long-grain rice – 37 per cent more than white long-grain rice
- wholewheat plain flour – 20 per cent more than white plain flour

- wholemeal self-raising flour – 51 per cent more than white self-raising flour
- sliced wholemeal bread – 15 per cent more than sliced white bread.

Take heart, though, because as products become more widely used, the price differential is reduced. For example, wholemeal bread (with a high turnover) is only 15% more expensive than white bread. This trend is likely to follow with other wholegrain food.

Don't forget that beans and lentils are a good source of fibre and starchy carbohydrate and these are about a third of the price of meat pound for pound.

Some nuts are better value than others. Peanuts make a good buy and hazelnuts can be quite reasonable. Buying them in large quantities usually saves quite a lot of money, but don't buy more than a few months' supply.

Vegetables and fruits are nearly always cheapest in a market, farm shop or at a greengrocer with a fast turnover. Try to plan your shopping so the greengrocery items can be bought separately from the other groceries. Naturally, freshness is an important factor. It is no good buying your vegetables and fruit weekly at a reasonable price if the source is not very fresh. You could find yourself throwing things away after a couple of days. Some of our research participants found that their food bills went down when changing their eating habits; this was because they relied more on home-grown fruits and vegetables. So if you have the chance to grow your own, this could save you money. In addition, the exercise taken out of doors will benefit your health and you will probably enjoy eating your own things more, simply because you have grown them.

Find out whether there is a wholefood co-operative in your area. Such an organisation is set up to help people who buy a lot of certain products within a given area. Bulk buying brings down the price and such ventures are usually run on a non-profit basis which further reduces costs. You can save a lot of money in this way, especially if you eat a lot of the particular foods they sell.

Storing Your High-fibre Foods

Some bread, cakes and buns are not date-marked because it is assumed they will be eaten within 24 hours of purchase. Store these in a cool, dry place. It is not surprising to learn that some bread manufacturers who need to keep bread fresh for prolonged periods (for example for ready-made packaged sandwiches) add extra fat to the bread. This is hardly a trend to be encouraged, especially as the fat is not polyunsaturated. However, some people do find the wholemeal bread goes a little drier after the first 24 hours. This can be overcome by keeping it wrapped in cling-film. Toasting wholemeal bread 3–4 days old, or warming in an oven usually gives good results. What you'll find though once you start eating a lot more fibre is that your bread consumption will go up so much that it won't have a chance to go stale. A family of four could be expected to eat at least a large wholemeal loaf within two days.

Wholegrain cereals and flours do not normally keep as long as refined ones. This is because the oil in the germ can oxidise with keeping and then taste rancid. Grains bought loose in a wholefood shop may not be date stamped. Most of these should keep fairly well if they are stored in a cool, dry place. Don't plan to keep them longer than six months. Dried peas, beans and lentils have good keeping qualities, provided they too are kept in a cool, dry place where air circulates. They may not be date-marked as many keep longer than eighteen months. Apart from being economical and a valuable part of a healthy diet, pulses are also good foods to have as a standby. They are even more useful to households without a freezer.

Vegetables too should be stored in a cool, dry place with some air circulating. The refrigerator dehydrates foods, so if you are using it to store vegetables or fruits, make sure they are covered, preferably with perforated plastic film or bags. Vegetables in sealed plastic bags can collect water and then start to rot. Vegetables and fruits are frequently sold in plastic bags rather than paper. Vegetables not stored in the fridge, such as potatoes, carrots, apples or oranges, which are sold in plastic bags should be transferred to paper ones for storage.

The following vegetables if bought fresh and stored correctly, should all keep for at least a week: celery, carrots, hard cabbage, fennel, Chinese leaf, Cos and Webb's lettuces in the summer, radishes, chicory, aubergine, courgettes.

Vegetables that will keep longer include: potatoes, parsnips, turnips, swede and onions. However, you should eat all vegetables as fresh as possible. They taste better and contain more vitamins when fresh.

Using a Freezer

For those who cannot shop regularly for fresh vegetables, frozen ones make a good alternative. Check how long you can store the vegetables (or fruit) in your particular fridge ice compartment or freezer. This is indicated by a star rating on the frozen food and on your fridge.

A freezer can be useful for storing wholemeal breads and wholemeal buns and scones, particularly if they are difficult to find in your locality. You may want to bake large batches of these, choosing a recipe that uses little sugar and fat. Make sure that all foods are frozen in airtight plastic bags. Once frozen, breads and buns do not keep fresh for as long when defrosted; this is because frozen foods lose moisture. You may find it helpful to cut a large loaf in half so you can just defrost enough for a day. The amount of bread you eat should increase on the new diet, so if you do have a freezer you will probably find it particularly useful for keeping reserves of different breads.

Dried beans can be cooked in a large batch and frozen ready for use in casseroles or salads. Try not to overcook them when they are for freezing as they may lose their shape.

Special Cooking Hints for Preparing High-fibre Foods

Vegetables and fruits

Clean off dirt and blemishes and remove insects; scrub skins. Try not to soak vegetables in water, particularly after cutting or bruising – this causes a loss of vitamins and minerals by leaching out into the water.

Whenever possible do not remove the skins as these provide

fibre and often minerals and vitamins are concentrated just under the skin. There is no need to remove plum and apple skins when making a crumble or pie.

Use as many of the well-washed outer leaves of vegetables as possible.

Try to eat vegetables or salad at least twice a day.

Cooked vegetables should be boiled in the minimum of water for the minimum of time.

Baked or casseroled vegetables are a good idea, but eaten with the cooking juice, as are steamed vegetables and vegetables lightly stir-fried in a very little polyunsaturated oil, ideally in a wok or non-stick pan.

Pulses

Wash. Most need soaking over 12 hours in three times their volume of cold water. Avoid adding salt as this toughens them and extends the cooking time. Don't cook beans in a slow cooker unless you have boiled them vigorously for more than 10 minutes beforehand.

Tinned pulses can be convenient but they are often canned in salty, sugary water and cost more. Savings on fuel, however, could cancel out the extra cost. See the chart on cooking beans, peas and lentils.

Rice

Wholegrain rice takes 5–10 minutes longer to cook than white rice.

Adding salt lengthens the time, so if you need to, add just a little salt once it is cooked.

Pasta and Flours

Wholewheat pasta takes just a little longer than white.

Wholegrain flours usually need more liquid when used for baking, but handle as little as possible. A little extra baking powder may help the raising, as will selecting recipes with an egg or yeast.

If you are used to cooking with white flour it may be helpful to start with 85 per cent extraction flour or a mixture of half white, half wholemeal. When you have gained confidence move on to 100 per cent wholewheat.

Extra-fine wholemeal flours can be found and these are useful when making wholemeal cakes.

Nuts

These can be used in a variety of ways – ground, chopped or whole. There is no need to blanch almonds or peanuts. The outer husk (not the shell) can be used.

High-fibre Dishes to Choose

Interesting Salads

Mixed vegetables in season, grated or sliced: red or white cabbage; sprouts; carrots; swede; raw beetroot; turnips; onion; green and red peppers; mushrooms; celery; fennel; chicory; courgettes, marrow and leek, lightly-cooked; or sprigs of cauliflower or beansprouts.

Add lemon juice, orange juice, vinegar, natural yoghurt or a little soya or corn oil for a dressing. Herbs, seeds like caraway, sunflower and sesame, chopped nuts, dried and fresh fruits all make tasty additions.

Cold wholegrain rice and pasta salads can make a pleasant change, as can salads with beans, both the dried ones and green beans, lightly-cooked and cooled.

Lettuce, cucumber and tomato can be made more exciting when cut into different shapes and mixed with onion, herbs, seeds and a vinegar dressing.

Cooked Vegetables

Don't bore your taste buds with plain boiled cabbage, carrots or peas. Try stuffed baked vegetables, such as potatoes, peppers, marrows, cabbage leaves or large mushrooms. Also try casseroled vegetables – red cabbage casserole or leek and potato casserole.

Stir-fried vegetables can be delicious. Good examples are shredded carrot, cabbage, onion, garlic and beansprouts and green pepper when they are in season. These can be mixed with cooked chicken or nuts. Vegetables can also be cooked in meat, fish or bean casseroles and in curries. They are useful in making the dish go further.

Pasta Dishes
Wholewheat pasta is a useful base for many quick, hot meals. Use different types for variety, e.g. spaghetti, macaroni, tubes, shells, rings etc. Onions, garlic, tomato, pepper, herbs or spinach can be added to give the base for a tasty dish and mixed with grated cheese, low-fat soft cheese, tinned and fresh fish, shellfish, lean mince (with the excess fat drained off before serving), cooked beans or lentils, nuts or finely-chopped lean ham.

Pasta can also be added to soups, used for puddings and is delicious cold in salads.

Rice
Long-grain wholegrain rice can be used as an addition to soups, casseroles and curries; to stuff vegetables and form the basis of a risotto or salad.

Short-grain or pudding rice can be used in puddings such as milk puddings with fruit.

Flours and Other Grains
Cracked wheat, or bulgar as it is also called, soaked for 1–2 hours is useful in soups, vegetable roasts or bakes and in salads.

Flaked cereals such as barley, rye, wheat, oats (sometimes called jumbo oats), make good toppings for savoury dishes and for fruit crumbles. Use them to replace some of the flour. They can also be added to meat, lentil and nut loaves. When making porridge try barley, rye or wheat flakes as a change from oats. These cereals, cooked whole, also make a delicious alternative to rice as an accompaniment to curries and casseroles.

Wholemeal flour makes a superb crumble mix. (Reduce the fat and sugar from the traditional recipes, see the recipes on page 198). It makes good scones, griddle cakes, breads, pizza bases and many other cakes. Cakes made by the creaming method are better when made with a fine wholemeal flour. Biscuits too bake well with wholegrain flours and with added, possibly flaked, wholegrains.

Nuts

These can be used to make rissoles, roasted nut loaves (bake as a meat loaf, but with nuts in place of meat). They can be eaten for snacks, alone or with dried fruit, added to salads, risottoes, vegetable curries and fruit salads.

Nut butters make good sandwich fillings and are popular with children. Try to choose those without added sugar, salt and oil.

Cooking Beans, Peas and Lentils

Soak beans for a minimum of 12 hours. Boil them vigorously for ten minutes before leaving them to simmer. The following are recommended cooking times:

Aduki beans	1 hour
Black beans	2 hours
Black-eyed beans	45 minutes
Butter beans or lima beans	1 hour
Chick peas	3 hours
Haricot beans	2 hours
Lentils (no soaking needed)	45 minutes–1 hour
Mung (or moong) beans	45 minutes
Pinto beans	1½ hours
Red kidney beans	1 hour
Split peas (no soaking needed)	1 hour
Soya beans	3-4 hours

The cooking times given are simply a guide. Some beans may take a little longer to become soft. In some cases you may want to reduce the simmering time a little and then cook the beans for a further period in a casserole in the oven. Alternatively, simmering may be continued a little longer with the addition of other vegetables and flavourings. If using a slow cooker, all beans (after soaking) should be boiled vigorously for 10 minutes on the stove before being slow-cooked.

Eating Out and Going Away

Wholemeal bread is much more widely available than it used to be. This is probably the easiest food with a high-fibre content to find when eating out. Choosing wholemeal sandwiches or rolls, a ploughman's lunch with wholemeal bread or soup with a wholemeal roll, all make good choices. If you only eat out or visit friends very occasionally, then there's no problem with eating what is on offer. However, many people eat out or visit the same take-away several times a week. In this case, if wholemeal bread is not available it is worth asking whether they could supply it. Then make a point of choosing the wholemeal bread and advertise the fact to your friends.

Baked beans, baked potatoes, salads and cooked vegetables are also quite easy to find, but wholegrain rice and pasta, wholemeal pizzas and wholemeal puddings are much more difficult to come by. Special wholefood and vegetarian cafés and restaurants are designed for those who enjoy high-fibre foods. There are paperback guide books of these cafés and restaurants. You may find you are lucky in your area.

It is worth asking in your canteen or local café if they will use wholemeal flour and serve wholegrain rice and pasta. After all, if you don't ask, they won't know there is any demand.

When you are staying away from home, breakfast may be a good meal at which to get your fibre and plenty of starchy carbohydrate. Choose a wholegrain or a high-fibre breakfast cereal and wholemeal rolls or toast. Fill up on these rather than a cooked breakfast, except tomatoes and mushrooms if they are offered, and also fruit. Many guest houses and hotels will get wholemeal bread in for you if you ask in advance, unless, of course, they normally supply it.

Once you get used to eating a lot of fibre and plenty of complex carbohydrate, you will probably find that you miss them when you go away. You may find you soon become constipated. This can be remedied by taking unprocessed bran with you and adding it to fruit juice or breakfast cereal. This occasional use of bran as a sort of 'medicine' makes good sense. You may also find you feel hungry when you are eating more refined, less bulky food. Those who put on weight easily will probably have to put up with feeling a little emptier than usual, otherwise eating refined foods, which are more concentrated in calories, until you feel full, will increase your weight. Topping up with fruit in between meals can be a way around this.

Fibre, Starchy Carbohydrate and Children

It is best to start children off on wholemeal bread rather than white right from the word go. Baby feeding will be discussed in terms of the whole diet later in the chapter. It is, however, relevant to make two points here. One is that wholemeal bread, toasted or baked in the oven, makes cheaper and less messy rusks for babies – they are also low in sugar. Second, children under 3 years should not be given chopped or whole nuts in case they choke.

Fresh and dried fruits make a good treat for children, particularly when presented in finger-sized pieces. Serve raw vegetables as a colourful platter of finger-sized pieces too. Cooked vegetables can be encouraged by making an expedition to your local greengrocers or market stall. Let the children choose the vegetables for the next meal and join in the cooking.

Similarly, wholemeal cakes, buns and biscuits made with a wholegrain flour and less sugar and fat than in traditional recipes can be prepared with the children. They will be eager to try them if they have helped to make them.

Many high-fibre foods make good snacks for children, particularly when they arrive home from school starving. You will find suggestions in the section on between-meals snacks (page 167).

A word of warning, don't suddenly change young children to a high-fibre diet. This can cause a sense of being bloated, stomach aches and diarrhoea, or very frequent motions. This will certainly turn them against what are very healthy foods.

Increasing the Fibre and Starchy Food in Your Diet

- Look through the shopping list of high-fibre and starchy foods. Pick out one or two that you could try or buy extra of them when you next go shopping.
- Introduce a few new high-fibre products into your normal recipes.
- As you decrease the fat and sugar in your diet, gradually serve more bread and larger portions of potato, rice and pasta.
- When you feel more adventurous, try new recipes with pulses, pasta, rice or wholegrain cereals.
- Increase fibre gradually, particularly with children, or if you are elderly. Increase your fluid intake at the same time.
- Balance the increased costs of the unrefined foods by cutting out the unnecessary or lavishly-packaged desserts, confectionery, pies and cakes. You will find it just about balances out.
- Dwell on the benefits of eating plenty of fibre – freedom from constipation, a feeling of fullness after a meal, plenty of food on the plate, and perhaps even the freedom to eat some of the foods you previously (and quite unjustly) thought were too fattening.

Are You Sweet Enough Already?
Eating Less Sugar

What is Sugar?

When we think of sugar it is generally the white substance, sucrose, which is added to tea, coffee and breakfast cereals and used in making sweets, cakes and biscuits. But sucrose is only one of a whole family of sugars. This includes fructose, glucose (dextrose), glucose syrup, maltose, honey, molasses and brown sugars. None of these sugars has any useful nutritional value apart from providing energy and you can get all the energy you need from other foods. Some sugars are found naturally in foods, such as fruits, vegetables and cereals. All of these are valuable foods. It is therefore the sugars added (often unnecessarily) to foods that you will need to reduce if you want to follow the NACNE guidelines. This means buying fewer bags of sugar as well as having less sugar, including honey, from sweets, cakes, biscuits, soft drinks and preserves.

Where Does the Sugar in our Diet Come From?

Sugar is widely distributed through many of the foods we eat. The table on pages 119 to 120 shows which foods contain most – you will probably be surprised at some of the foods which you may have thought were sugar-free.

How to Eat Less Sugar

- Cut down on sugar taken in drinks and in cooking.
- Choose foods with a lower-sugar content in preference to foods high in added sugar.

Lower-sugar choice	High-sugar choice
Nuts and raisins, grapes, dried fruit	Sweets and chocolates
Plain biscuits, crispbreads*, bread, rolls, home-made fruit breads and scones without jam	Chocolate, cream-filled and iced biscuits
Banana, apple etc	Cakes, sweet pastries
Cottage and curd cheeses*, quark, peanut butter*, paste*, natural all-fruit preserve with no added sugar	Jam, honey, marmalade, lemon curd, chocolate spread
Fresh, dried and stewed fruit, fruit tinned in natural juice with natural yoghurt or buttermilk. Milk puddings or	Tinned fruit in syrup, flavoured yoghurts, jelly, ice-cream. Other puddings and desserts

Low-sugar choice	High-sugar choice
fruit crumble made with little or no sugar	
Pickled vegetables*, e.g. onions, gherkins	Sweet pickles*, ketchup and fruit sauces*
Diluted pure fruit juice, water, soda or carbonated water*	Fizzy drinks and squash, including 'health' drinks, containing sugar

*These are also high in salt

Make a big effort to reduce sugary snacks and sweet drinks between meals.

How Much Sugar do the High-sugar Choices Contain?

This information has been taken from an article in the *Journal of Human Nutrition 1978, Vol. 32*, pages 335–47 by D. A. T. Southgate – the journal that most dietitians read.

Really what we want to know is *all* the sugar, but there is no reliable source for this information. This table, therefore, includes just the sucrose which, in most cases, is the *added* sugar. Where a value is given in brackets ( ), this means the total sugar in the food has been included because nearly all of it is added.

The Sugar in Food

	Sugar content (in g) per 100g of food	How much is 100g?	Sugar content in teaspoons
Drinking chocolate	73.8	2/5ths of small tin	15
Plain chocolate	58.7	One 100g bar	12
Sugar Puffs	45.6	3 helpings	9

Continued	Sugar content (in g) per 100g of food	How much is 100g?	Sugar content in teaspoons
Fully coated fancy chocolate biscuit	38.2	About 5 biscuits	8
Fruit cake	35.5	Large slice	7
Ginger nuts	32.8	Half a small pkt.	6½
Half coated chocolate digestive	26.0	Half a small pkt.	5
Fruit pie	21.5	One small to medium sized portion	4
Sweet Vermouth	(15.9)	1/10th of a litre bottle	3
Dry Vermouth	(5.5)	1/10th of a litre bottle	1
Ice-cream – non-dairy	(15.4)[1]	2 small scoops	3
All-Bran	12.1	3 helpings	2½
Fruit yoghurt	10.2	2/3rds of a carton	2
Cola drink	10.1	1/3rd of a can	2
Canned strawberries	7.0 (21.1)	Half a small can	1½
Tinned rice pudding	5.1	¼ of a tin	1
Baked beans	3.4	Less than a ¼ of a standard sized can	1
Fresh strawberries	1.1 (5.9)[2]	One helping	– (1)[2]
Shredded Wheat	negligible	–	–

[1]this is added sucrose and glucose but not total sugar
[2]this is all naturally-occurring

Reprinted by courtesy of John Libbey & Co. Ltd.

What About Artificial Sweeteners?

Artificial sweeteners such as saccharin, aspartame and acesulfame K are all permitted additives. Their availability makes it easier to achieve a reduction in sugar in a population which, by and large, is addicted to sweetness. This is particularly true when sugar is used just for sweetening such as in soft drinks, rather than to provide texture as in a toffee.

There are, however, drawbacks to their use. You may find they leave an aftertaste in the mouth. In the case of saccharin some people complain of a bitter aftertaste. This is especially true after boiling. For example, when stewing fruit, saccharin should be added after cooking. Aspartame and acesulfame K may have less of an aftertaste, but they are several times more expensive, and using any of these replacements for sugar does not educate your palate to enjoy less sweet foods. Problems arise when products cannot be made easily without sugar, such as jams, sweets and cakes or when an artificially sweetened product you are used to is not available. There is another school of thought that is concerned that although these sweeteners help reduce tooth decay they might be harmful in other respects. Some experts claim that it is less hazardous to health to eat a little sugar than to eat any of these artificial sweeteners on the basis that sugar is at least a natural, if refined, product.

Artificial sweeteners come under the Food and Drugs Act and are controlled by the Minister of Agriculture, Fisheries and Food and the Secretary of State for Social Services. These ministers are advised by the Food Advisory Committee which in turn obtains evidence from interested parties and the public as well as from other specialist advisory committees of the Department of Health and Social Security. The need for an additive must first be established and its safety tested before it can be used in foods. New research findings on additives are continuously assessed. This is also true in the case of artificial sweeteners.

Aspartame is known to be unsafe for people (mainly children) suffering from the rare condition phenylketonuria. The Food Additives and Contaminants Committee Report *The Review of Sweeteners in Food* (HMSO 34 1982) states that 'there is no reason to review the current use of saccharin' and that 'recent studies have failed to show an increased incidence in cancer'.

At the moment research is confused on the subject so you really need to make up your own mind whether you wish to take artificial sweeteners at all, to limit their use or to use them freely to replace sugar in the foods you eat. A sensible approach is to try and reduce the number of sweet foods you eat and to use artificial sweeteners for a few foods when it suits you.

This is also a sensible approach with children. Drinking a few artificially-sweetened soft drinks is probably inevitable, but by choosing sugar-free varieties you will help to preserve your children's teeth. Limiting other sweet foods will help prevent a sweeth tooth from developing.

Using Artificial Sweeteners

Artificial sweeteners come in tablet, liquid and powder forms. Read the labels to see what you are buying. Many of them are part sugar, so don't be misled. Liquid sweetener can be useful for sweetening cooked fruit or for adding to milk or other liquids. The tablets are best used in hot drinks where they dissolve. Powdered sweeteners can be sprinkled on to or into most drinks and foods, but they do not have the structure of sugar which is often required for baking.

Shopping for Less Sugar

Reduced-sugar drinks are now much more widely available. The following low- or reduced-sugar products can be found in most large supermarkets:

Unsweetened fruit juice
Tinned fruit in natural juice
Low-calorie fruit squash (but containing some sugar)
Low-calorie fizzy drinks (may contain sugar)
Low-calorie mixers (mostly containing some sugar)
Reduced-sugar or 'extra' jams and marmalades
Savoury biscuits (although these may be high in salt as well as fat)
Oat cakes
Crispbreads
Scones, muesli bread, currant bread (avoid those with a sticky glazed top – on the whole these are less sweet than other cakes)

Unsweetened breakfast cereals, e.g. Shredded Wheat, unsweetened muesli
Fresh and dried fruits
Natural and fruit yoghurts without added sugar

Reduced-sugar preserves may in fact be a waste of money; they frequently come in smaller jars and, allowing for this, can be 50 per cent more expensive than the ordinary versions. In some cases there is only 15 per cent more fruit in the lower-sugar version. It might make more sense simply to cut down on the amount of ordinary jam you use. To have a larger choice of reduced-sugar foods you will probably need to visit a health food or wholefood store. However, you can easily achieve the NACNE goal set for sugar by eating a somewhat simpler diet which involves limiting cakes and biscuits and processed manufactured foods containing sugar. You do not need to search for the specialist low-sugar products sold at premium prices. We hope that in time they will become available in supermarkets at a reasonable price.

You may find some of the following products in a wholefood or health food store:

Reduced-sugar confectionery
Lower-sugar biscuits
Oatcakes
Sugar-free baked beans
Low-sugar ketchup
Peanut butter with no added sugar
All fruit preserves – with no added sugar
Fruit spread made from concentrated fruit juices

These last two items are very high in natural sugar and in the case of the spread, the skin and pips which provide fibre have been removed. As they have a strong fruit taste, less can be used than ordinary preserves.

In the case of jams you may find the reduced-sugar version is also free from colourings and preservatives. When thinking about cost, weigh up whether this is important to you.

You will probably have to visit a chemist to obtain the following:

Artificial sweeteners
Sugar-free sweets, e.g. sugar-free gums
Sugar-free fruit squashes, e.g. diabetic.

Some products can contain sorbitol and be labelled low-sugar. These are usually marketed for diabetics. Sorbitol is just as high in energy as sugar but is more slowly absorbed by the body. If too much is taken at a time, diarrhoea can result.

Reading the Labels

When thinking about consuming less sugar, do read the ingredient labels. It is very easy to be deceived. Look and see where sugar comes on the ingredient list or, if stated, how much sugar the food contains. Remember, all the following terms mean sugar has been added: sucrose, lactose, fructose, glucose, glucose syrup, dextrose, syrup, maltose, honey, brown sugar, raw cane sugar, molasses.

Many fruit squashes and fizzy drinks contain sugar but less than half that of ordinary soft drinks. The squashes free of added sugar which are suitable for diabetics may contain more fruit juices than the low-calorie ones which contain sugar. They therefore cost a little more. Some confectionery advertised as 'low-sugar' or 'no added sugar' may contain honey, glucose or fructose. Some fruit juices have sugar added and other fruit drinks sold in cartons, looking like unsweetened fruit juices, contain large amounts of sugar. Here you will need to read labels very carefully.

Most muesli is marketed with a healthy image. Make up your own mind by reading the label. Many brands sold in supermarkets contain brown sugar. Also check which other breakfast cereals do not contain sugar and then select the sugar-free ones that you like.

Some products may contain more than one kind of sugar. They will be entered more than once on the label.

What About Price?

Reducing your intake of sugary foods saves money. Confectionery, chocolate biscuits and soft drinks all carry VAT. They are therefore relatively expensive. Individual cream desserts and cakes are expensive too. Keeping to basic foods which are lower in sugar is cheaper. Where you could run into extra cost is buying special reduced-sugar products or fresh fruits out of season. However, the money saved on other sweet foods will allow you to buy a few of these non-essential but special products or other treats such as dried fruits, nuts or exotic fresh fruits. Low-calorie squashes containing a little sugar are often cheaper than normal whole-fruit drinks, but don't forget that water is the cheapest and most thirst-quenching drink of all. The following price differentials were noted in a large supermarket:

- low-calorie squash (containing some sugar) – 25 per cent cheaper than ordinary whole-fruit drink
- sugar-free whole-fruit drink – 2 per cent more than ordinary whole-fruit drink
- low-calorie fizzy drinks and mixers – same price as ordinary ones
- tinned fruit in natural juice – up to 20 per cent more than the same fruit tinned in syrup (but shop around if you can)
- all-fruit preserves (from a health food store) – 200 per cent more than ordinary jam
- low-sugar baked beans (from a health food store) – 165 per cent more than ordinary baked beans.

Storing Your Low-sugar Groceries

Fresh fruits are best stored in a cool place with the air circulating and once ripe, eaten as quickly as possible. Freezing a surplus picked in the garden or bought cheaply when in season makes sense. Follow a freezer book for advice on blanching the fruit. For other non-perishable goods store according to the storage instructions on the label and don't buy more than you will need before the 'best before' date is reached. Most long-life fruit juices and soft drinks keep, unopened, in good condition for a few months. Tinned and dried fruits keep well when stored properly because the natural sugar they contain acts as a preservative. A lower-sugar diet should not pose any problems to keeping an adequate food store. The main precaution is to refrigerate reduced-sugar preserves once they are opened. Home-made jams and chutneys made with less sugar are also best kept in the fridge. In warm weather low-sugar cakes and buns are best stored in the fridge.

Asking for Low-sugar Foods

As you get used to foods that are less sweet you will find most of the proprietary foods too sweet and you may not have time to make your own lower-sugar versions. As with the higher-fibre products you would like to see, let the supermarket manager or manufacturer know that you would prefer less sugar in your baked beans or less sugar in your biscuits. If enough people make the same request, he will respond as their profits depend on what you, the consumer, will buy.

You may find in some foreign countries that drinks come ready sweetened. You need to think ahead and order your drinks without sugar. You may need to behave in the same way in this country when ordering fresh grapefruit or other fresh fruits.

Taking Less Sugar at Home

Breakfast
- Choose unsweetened fruit juice rather than sweetened.
- Choose unsweetened breakfast cereal and leave the sugar off the table.
- Use a little less jam or marmalade or use one with less sugar. Alternatively, use peanut butter or a low-fat soft cheese with bread or toast.

● Take unsweetened tea or coffee (artificially sweetened if necessary to start with).

Main meals
● Choose simpler puddings.
● Unsweetened fruit either fresh, dried and reconstituted (rehydrated) or tinned in natural juice. Have natural yoghurt for a change or, for a treat, have chopped nuts or seeds on top.
● When making a more substantial pudding, choose something like wholemeal bread and butter pudding. Add dried fruit and, if necessary, an artificial sweetener.
● Wholemeal crumble can be made with half the sugar most recipes recommend. Also avoid adding sugar to the fruit.
● Milk puddings can be made using a reduced-fat milk and sweetened with dried fruit or an artificial sweetener.

Between-Meals Snacks

This can be the hardest time to reduce sugar, but the most important. Sugar can do even more harm to the teeth when taken frequently between meals rather than taken all in one go at a meal. Suggestions for suitable in-between-meal snacks are included in the snack section at the end of the chapter. When you feel like cakes or buns choose the lower-sugar ones which are suggested in that section, but when possible, choose the other sugar-free suggestions. The recipe for apple and raisin teabread is an example of a suitable low-sugar teatime food to bake. With most recipes you can at least halve the sugar content, giving excellent results, with the exception of Swiss roll, sponge, meringues, Victoria sandwich, sweets and royal icing. Griddle cakes can be made with little sugar if dried fruit is added. Also, home-made biscuits need only very little added sugar. Remember not to sprinkle icing sugar or brush a sugar syrup on to baked foods – they are not necessary.

Limiting Sugar When Eating Out or Going Away

In most places, sugar is the easiest of the NACNE goals to achieve when eating away from home. It is usually quite possible to avoid a dessert or to choose fruit and of course you don't have to add sugar to your food at the table. If you don't eat out often then selecting a sweet pudding or cake when you do is not really important. When you eat out often, then you do need to think about the sugar. You may feel hungry if you avoid desserts, but this can be prevented by filling up on potatoes, bread, rice or pasta in your first course. In the case of many school cafeterias or school dinners it can be difficult to choose an adequately filling meal that is low in sugar. Just a piece of fruit for pudding can mean your child is starving by mid-afternoon. Advise them on the savoury foods to fill up on, or pack a filling lunch.

When regularly visiting friends who offer sweet foods, be brave and refuse if you don't really want them. They will go on offering, and coaxing you to have some if you do accept them each time.

Nuts and raisins or fresh fruit will make a good replacement for sweets if you find you must nibble something when you are travelling.

Children and Sugar

Children don't miss what they have never had. It can be much harder for adults to reduce their sugar when they have become accustomed to sweet foods. Children do not necessarily always go for the sweet foods; they go for finger-sized foods, and may like savoury things much more than sugary ones. It just so happens that in most cases sweet foods are finger-sized. Don't let your children start the habit of having sugar in drinks or added to cereals, then they will never miss it. Soft drinks should be thought of as a treat, not as an everyday food. Water is a natural drink and leaves you money to spend on something better. It is worth remembering that a can of Coca-Cola contains roughly seven teaspoons of sugar, yet few children drink it because they are hungry.

Sweets are unnecessary – healthy children can get all the energy they need from better food. Having said this, there is no need to ban sweets. It is not that sugar is poisonous or directly harmful other than to teeth. It is the total effect of eating too much sugar and then having insufficient of other nutrients valuable for health. When taken in excess it can also lead to overweight. It is better to let your children eat sweets all in one go at a meal than to be sucking them on and off all day. Most children grow up quite happily eating fruit as a daily treat if they are brought up this way from the start.

If you are used to icing cakes for children, try decorating them with nuts and dried fruits in colourful and exciting patterns, or with their name or age. Some children prefer this to 'boring' icing.

When your children go out to friends, let them have what the other children eat. They may not want the sweet foods even if they are offered. When other children come to you, avoid the sugary drinks, sweets and sticky cakes and biscuits. Use the occasion to help them to see that there is a better way to eat which can still be tasty and fun.

Adjusting to Less Sugar

The participants in our Study, on the whole, found the sugar goal quite easy to achieve. No doubt many had read so much about sugar over the years that they had educated their palates to enjoy less sweet foods and found this goal no hardship. Many of the participants offered their advice on how to cut down on sugar.

● Remember that it is everyday habits that count. Try gradually to wean yourself off the practice of adding sugar to drinks, cereals and fruits. You will reach a point when you won't want the sugar on the table and it may be difficult to find it when requested by a guest.

● Think of cakes and rich puddings as a Sunday treat or for special occasions. Cakes, buns and biscuits with less sugar (and fat) can be delicious and just as much of a treat. You may have time to make them if you don't need them every day.

• Use an artificial sweetener as a way of weaning yourself off sugar, but have fewer sweet foods generally as your goal.

• Try not to let yourself get over-hungry or tired as this can set off the desire for sweet foods – yet they won't satisfy you for long. Eat sufficient of the high-fibre, starchy foods to prevent you feeling hungry between meals.

• Eat sweet foods at a meal rather than in between meals. This is particularly important for children. Sugary foods, apart from harming teeth can reduce the appetite for more nutritious foods. This is why they have been called 'empty calories'.

• Allow yourself an occasional, controlled binge on sweet foods. A craving once in a while may be quite natural. Women, in particular, may feel like sweets and chocolates towards the end of their menstrual cycle. If this is true for you try to plan your healthy way of eating to include this. Banning something sweet at this time might build up to your eating far more of other things than you otherwise would. It might be helpful to keep a chocolate bar, biscuit or choc-ice – whatever appeals to you, ready for this time of the month.

• Cutting down on sugary foods does save money, so think of a treat you can have instead, such as an outing or an exotic fruit, vegetable or fish.

• Remember, cakes, biscuits, sugary drinks and sweets were never meant to be a main source of food. Unfortunately, millions of people treat them as such today and it is they who are at real risk from the massive sugar load they consume.

• Cutting children down on daily or frequent rations of sweets can be difficult once the habit is established. The best way is to put the money in a jar and let the children see it grow. Make sure they have something they are saving for. This approach can help adults as well. In some families one child may be more like one parent and gain weight or get tooth decay easily, whereas another does not. It is much better to treat all the family the same and have few sweets in the house. One of the best possible ways of helping the sweet problem is to have no sweets at all in the house but to have a once-a-week 'sweet day' during which the children are allowed to eat a fixed ration of sweets, preferably of their choice. This will keep small children going for the whole week (together with the anticipation!).

Full of Fitness not Fatness: Eating Less Fat

Which Fats are the Problem?

The fat we eat is not only in easily visible forms such as butter, margarine and cooking oils. There is a lot of hidden fat in food too. In fact about five-eighths of our fat comes in a hidden form from meat, meat products, milk, cheese, cream, eggs, chocolates, cakes, biscuits, pastries and other convenience foods. When thinking about cutting down on fats it is the *total* fat in your diet that you should be aiming to control.

To some extent it is a matter of deciding which habits are the least important to you. You may find it easy to cut down on butter, margarine, cooking fats, and the fat in milk (by changing to a lower-fat milk). Alternatively, you may prefer to cut down on your meat products, full-fat cheese, biscuits and pastries.

Although the goal should be to reduce the total amount of fat, your priority should be to eat less of the saturated fats. These fats come from animals and some vegetables such as coconut and palm, and are hard at room temperature. Some saturated fats are found when vegetable oils have been hardened during the manufacture of margarines. When choosing which habits to change bear in mind that the fat you least want comes from meat, cheese, butter, lard, milk, meat products and most high-fat processed foods. Cutting down on saturated fats will reduce the total amount of fat you eat. In addition it will raise the proportion of polyunsaturated fats compared with the saturated.

Polyunsaturated fats are mainly of vegetable origin (some come from oily fish) and are oily or soft at room temperature. You can also help to raise the proportion of polyunsaturated fats in your diet by only cooking with an oil made from corn, soya or sunflower seeds. Blended vegetable oils are not as good as they contain more saturated fat. Or you could use a margarine which states that it is high in polyunsaturated fat. The trouble with fat is that it is loaded with calories so if you gain weight easily be careful to use only a little oil and margarine even if it is labelled 'high in polyunsaturates, lower in saturates'. A margarine high in polyunsaturates is just as fattening as other margarines and butter and twice as high in calories as low-fat spreads.

What are the Main Sources of Fat in our Diet?

26 per cent comes from meat products
13 per cent comes from margarine
12 per cent from cooking fats
12 per cent comes from milk
11 per cent from butter
7 per cent from cheese and cream
6 per cent from biscuits/cakes and pastries
3 per cent from eggs
10 per cent from all other foods

How to Eat Less Fat

- Use only a little in cooking and spread less on bread.
- Choose foods with a lower-fat content to replace high-fat foods you normally eat.

Low-fat choice	High-fat choice
Foods cooked with little or no fat – grilled, baked, poached, casseroled, boiled, steamed	Foods cooked with fat – fried, roasted; gravy from the meat fat
Dried beans, split peas, lentils, baked beans*, fish, fish fingers*, chicken/turkey (no skin), rabbit, lean meat, offal	Fatty meat, tinned meat*, sausages*, burgers*, pasties*, meat pies*, salami*

Quark and cottage cheese* – the lowest; curd or low-fat hard cheeses*	Full-fat cheeses*: Cheddar, blue cheeses and Cheshire cream cheeses
Skimmed, semi-skimmed milk	Whole and evaporated milk
Buttermilk, low-fat yoghurt	Cream – dairy, soured, artificial; ice cream
Vinegar, lemon juice, yoghurt dressings	Mayonnaise, salad cream*
Boiled, baked and mashed potato	Chips, roast potatoes, crisps*
Potato or scone mixture for pie toppings	Pastry
Bread, crispbreads*, home-made scones, muffins, fruit breads and griddle cakes	Biscuits, cakes and pastries
Mixed nuts and dried fruit, raw vegetables e.g. carrots, celery	Chocolates, toffees, savoury snacks*: crisps, salted biscuits

*may be high in salt.

For fat in cooking, choose fats and oils high in polyunsaturated fat such as corn, soya or sunflower seed oil – but use sparingly.

What Sort of Differences are There Between High-fat and Low-fat Choices?

High-fat choice	% fat	Low-fat choice	% fat
Whole milk	4	Skimmed milk	Trace
Double cream	48	Low-fat yoghurt	1
Cheddar cheese	34	Cottage cheese	4
Chocolate cake	27	Bread	2
Chips	11*	Baked potato	Trace
Crisps	36	Orange/apple	Trace

Continued

High-fat choice	% fat	Low-fat choice	% fat
Fried white fish	10*	Steamed white fish	1
Streaky back bacon	40	Lean pork chop (excluding bone)	11
Butter and ordinary margarine	82	Low-fat spread	41

* Can be considerably higher than this.

Shopping for Less Fat

Fortunately, food manufacturers, dairies and supermarkets are responding by making more lower-fat foods available. But keeping fats down can be difficult when eating away from home. It is thus essential to take every opportunity when shopping to buy foods that are low in fat. A large supermarket is definitely the best place to find low-fat foods but all grocers will stock at least some of the foods to look out for. It is also worth remembering that the larger supermarkets may have a delicatessen section selling many high-fat foods, as well as a wide variety of rich cakes and biscuits. Whilst looking for the better foods, you may have to exercise self-control over these. Make sure these rich, high-fat foods only get into your basket on special occasions. When out shopping look for the following foods; some are naturally low in fat and some have had the fat removed.

Semi-skimmed/skimmed milk (if you can't get them from your milkman)
Natural, low-fat yoghurt
Low-fat soft cheese or quark
Edam, Gouda, Shape or Tendale or other medium-fat hard cheeses
Lean meat or offal
Chicken/Turkey (with the skin removed)
Rabbit
Fish – all kinds, fresh, frozen or tinned white and oily fish,

(smoked fish and some tinned fish is very high in salt)
Dried and canned beans, peas and lentils
Margarine high in polyunsaturates; or low-fat spread*
Corn, soya or sunflower oil*
Reduced-fat sausages
Lean mince
Plenty of breads, cereals, pasta and rice (to fill up on)
Currant breads and rolls, scones, malt loaf and Swiss roll
sponge (without a cream filling) – these are lower-fat cakes but
may be rather high in sugar
Low-calorie salad cream, salad dressing and mayonnaise
(these should be used sparingly as they are still quite high in
fat)
Thick-cut chips – just occasionally
* Although these are high sources of fat they are fine if used sparingly.

Your Milkman

Most dairies now bring to the door skimmed milk which has
only a trace of fat and semi-skimmed milk which has half the
fat of ordinary milk. There have been complaints that semi-
skimmed milk goes off too quickly. This is probably because
the demand has not been adequately assessed by the dairy. It
is not a problem which should continue.

Reading the Labels

Pressure by the public and those interested in food and health
is bringing about improvements in the labelling of food. This
will help you judge whether a particular food is high in fat and
whether most of the fat is saturated or not.

It *can* be difficult to find out exactly which fat or oil a food
contains. You may come across the terms vegetable oil, animal
fat, beef fat, pork fat, lard, suet, non-milk fat, or non-animal
fat. These last two terms confuse many people who then think
the food is low-calorie. They simply mean the fat is not from
milk and not from animals. Ice-creams, for example, may be
labelled 'non-milk fat'. This does not mean low-fat – they will
probably contain a vegetable oil. Similarly, some powdered

milks say 'skimmed milk powder' but if you read further you may find they have added vegetable oils, i.e. non-milk fats.

Asking for Low-fat Foods

This is a clear case where consumer demand has resulted in better availability of products – for example, in bringing low-fat milks to the doorstep and low-fat cheeses and spreads and reduced-fat sausages to the shops. Consumer pressure has also succeeded in making leaner fresh meat more widely available. Keep on asking for these things and you will find that the lower-fat milks become easier to find and that they will be fresher. Other lower-fat meat products will also become available. They may seem more expensive but remember that you can buy less as you won't be buying the unnecessary fat that is bulking out most of the current meat products.

What About Price?

At a first glance buying lower-fat foods may seem more expensive. But we are not suggesting that you make anything other than a very gradual change. Simply replacing meat pies and meat products with lean meat and fish could cost more. The message is really to eat less meat, and to choose the lean. When buying meat products such as pies and processed cold meats, you are buying a whole lot of fat you don't want. Using beans and lentils to replace some meat saves money.

The following price differentials were observed between high-fat foods and their lower-fat alternatives in a large supermarket (February 1985):

- butter cost 72 per cent more than margarine high in polyunsaturates (both were the shop's own brand)
- margarine high in polyunsaturates cost 35 per cent more than margarine high in saturated fat
- low-fat spread (own brand) cost 7 per cent more than margarine high in saturated fat and cost less than half the price of butter

- fresh skimmed milk 7 per cent cheaper than whole fresh milk
- lower-fat natural yoghurt 5 per cent cheaper than whole-milk yoghurt
- soya oil* cost 6 per cent more than blended vegetable oils
- lean braising beef cost 32 per cent more than fresh beef burgers
- pig's liver and kidneys cost 59 per cent less than fresh beef burgers
- orange lentils cost 68 per cent less than fresh beef burgers – weight for weight
- low-calorie mayonnaise and salad cream were found to be the same price as standard products.

*Soya oil is higher in polyunsaturates than a blended oil.

So you can see that some of the lower-fat choices cost more but others will save you money. When comparing lean beef and a beef burger don't forget that you need less of the lean beef (the extra fuel for cooking does, however, need to be taken into consideration). Lean mince costs more than standard mince but again you need considerably less so the cost evens out.

Remember that when you are buying a low-fat spread you are paying for extra water so if you are watching your pennies carefully it is better to buy a polyunsaturated margarine and to use it *very sparingly*. The participants in our study who used predominantly a low-fat spread were in fact eating just as much fat but were paying twice as much for it.

Storing Your Low-fat Foods

As with all food products, read the storage conditions on the fat-containing products you buy.

Low-fat spreads do not keep as well as the full-fat ones because of the extra water content. Only buy as much as you can expect to use by the 'best before' date. Low-fat soft cheeses do not keep for long so the same applies here. Always read the date stamp and buy the one with the latest date. Tinned fish and pulses (including baked beans) do keep well so these can make a good standby.

When fats and oils are kept too long they oxidise and go rancid. This is something to be aware of. You may, for example, find it necessary to buy smaller bottles of oil and tubs of margarine as you start to use less.

Preparing and Cooking Food with Less Fat

Having bought the foods that will help you eat a lower-fat diet you then need to think about how you can serve them in an enjoyable way – not forgetting, of course, that the way you cook your food can affect its fat content. For example, frying will increase the fat content. It can also be reduced by trimming all visible fat off meat, skimming it off the top of stews, and draining mince.

Useful Cooking Utensils for Low-fat Cookery
A good, deep non-stick frying pan is a great asset (together with non-stick utensils)
A wok (to add variety to your cooking)
Heavy cast-iron pans
A grill and grill pan

Meat
- Trim off visible fat
- Grill steak, chops and bacon
- Brown meat in its *own* fat in a non-stick pan or heavy cast-iron pan along with any vegetables used in the dishes – onions, garlic, peppers or other vegetables
- Use less meat and replace with more vegetables. Peas, beans and lentils can be used to replace some meat. Cook until nearly soft before adding to the meat dish, or use canned ones (remembering these have added salt and sugar).
- Mince can be very high in fat – never add fat when frying it – onions and vegetables can be browned with the mince fat. Drain the fat before serving.

- Make good use of tasty vegetables, e.g. tomatoes, celery, onions, garlic, peppers, mushrooms, herbs and spices so you don't miss the fat.
- Remove the skin from chicken and turkey as this is very fatty.
- Do not add fat when roasting meat. If you are worried about having dry meat it is better to pot roast (cook in the oven with little liquid under a tight lid).
- A slow cooker can be useful for making casseroles for the busy cook who would otherwise fry or heat up pies!
- When grilling – grill well and allow the fat to drip into the grill pan.
- Occasional frying is not completely taboo but use very hot fat and drain foods on absorbent kitchen paper before serving.
- A microwave can leave meat succulent and no fat is required.

Sauces and Dressings
- Thicken sauces with cornflour or plain flour rather than by making a fat and flour roux. Use semi-skimmed or skimmed milk.
- When using cheese in sauces and toppings choose a strongly-flavoured one and use less.
- Delicious dressings can be made for salads from yoghurt, vinegar, lemon juice and herbs or use a low-calorie dressing extended with yoghurt.
- Herbs, nuts and seeds can be added to give salads flavour.
- Vegetables cooked to a soft pulp or puréed make a good sauce or will thicken casseroles, gravies and soups.
- Yoghurt makes a good substitute for sour cream and is delicious with curries or baked potatoes. To avoid curdling, add after the food is removed from the heat.
- Buttermilk and yoghurt are good with fruit puddings.
- Curry spices have more flavour when cooked in a little fat so fry with the meat or add just a little oil to fry them in.

Vegetables

● Fried vegetables such as courgettes or aubergines can absorb lots of fat so try to use other methods of preparing them. They can be sweated in a lightly greased non-stick or cast-iron pan on a low heat. Tomatoes and garlic can be added and they taste much lighter and fresher than when fried.

● Baked or casseroled vegetables are tasty and don't require fat for cooking.

● Shredded and finely-sliced vegetables, cauliflower florets and beansprouts can be stir-fried in a lightly-greased wok.

● Avoid adding butter and margarine to cooked vegetables – if you want them moist cook them in a casserole or serve with a casserole.

● Cooking vegetables in the main dish to give you a 'one-pot meal' preserves the flavour (i.e.. it is not thrown down the sink in the cooking water), it also saves on fuel and cooking utensils. This also helps to extend a meat dish helping you to cut down on meat.

● Mash potato with milk instead of butter (use skimmed or semi-skimmed).

Avocados are naturally oily so don't serve with an oily dressing – lemon juice is much more suitable.

● When cooking bean or lentil dishes it is quite acceptable to use a little oil in which to brown onions or garlic or for cooking spices as beans contain so little fat.

● All chips are high in fat but it can be minimised by cutting them thickly and frying them quickly in very hot fat and draining them on a kitchen paper towel before serving.

Nuts

● Nuts contain quite a lot of fat so you should only need to add a little fat, if any at all, to a recipe that contains them (such as a nut roast).

Fish

● There are an infinite number of ways of cooking tasty fish dishes without frying or adding fat. Mackerel, herring, sardines and trout all grill beautifully without added fat.

- Fish fingers can be baked in the oven or grilled without adding fat.
- Fillets of fish can be just lightly greased and grilled after adding herbs and spices of your choice.
- Casseroled fish can be delicious with vegetables such as tomatoes, onions and garlic plus herbs, or with spinach.
- Fish also makes delicious curries – no fat is needed except a tablespoon of oil for frying the spices, onions and other vegetables gently.
- Tinned fish (drain the oil before using) – has a variety of uses: mixed into salads, served on its own in a salad, grilled on toast, baked in a casserole, added to rice or pasta.

Puddings and Pies
- Make puddings and pies occasional foods – with two-layer or enclosed pastry dishes a thing of the past. Put just one layer of pastry on top of fruit or meat pies or make open tarts.
- Use a fat or oil high in polyunsaturates for the pastry.
- Cut down on the fat used in fruit crumble and use more fruit. Extra wheat or other cereal flakes help to give crunch.
- Potato makes a good topping for savoury dishes instead of pastry – it can be mashed or cut into slices.
- Scone mixture or choux pastry makes a lower-fat topping than ordinary pastry – for savoury or fruit dishes.
- Bread pudding can be made without buttering the bread and using a low-fat milk. Use low-fat milks when making custard and milk puddings.
- A cheesecake for a special occasion can be made using a low-fat soft cheese, yoghurt and curd cheese rather than cream or cream cheese.

Savoury snacks
- There is no need to put fat on toast that is to be topped with beans, eggs, cheese, fish etc. Neither is it necessary to use fat on bread when a moist spread or filling is used: meat, cheese, nut butter etc.
- Just spread one side of a sandwich with fat. Scrambled egg can be cooked in a non-stick pan without fat using a little low-fat milk.

- Cook poached eggs without fat.
- Raw vegetables on their own or stuffed with dried fruit or low-fat soft cheese make good replacements for crisps and savoury biscuits.

Sweet Snacks
- Choose the lower-fat cakes and breads – there is no need to spread butter on to tea breads or malt loaves.
- Choose cake recipes that are low in fat – this means avoiding cakes made by creaming fat and sugar or by the rich, rubbed-in method.
- Lower-fat cakes and teabreads are quicker to make than the high-fat ones. Just use 30–55g fat to 250g wholemeal flour (1–2oz fat to 8oz flour).
- Griddle cakes can be made by cooking on a lightly-greased cast-iron surface.
- For cakes and biscuits which call for a rather high-fat content make sure you use a fat or oil high in polyunsaturates.

Detecting Fat
When preparing, cooking and serving food you can often detect how greasy it is. Observe whether the grease is left on the plate or separates out in the cooking pot on cooling. Greasy foods usually leave a greasy mark on a piece of kitchen roll and they feel greasy to the touch – pâté and sausage meat, for example. In many foods such as salami or black pudding, you can actually see the fat.

Low-fat Dishes and Foods to Choose at Home

Breakfast
- Plenty of cereal with low-fat milk
- Wholemeal bread with a little polyunsaturated fat or low-fat spread
- Fresh fruit

Main Meals

- Fish pie with fish in a low-fat white sauce (cornflour and low-fat milk) *or* fish plus tomatoes and onions topped with mashed potato
- Mixed bean and vegetable pie with potato topping
- Beef and bean curry with rice
- Tuna fish, sweetcorn and peas mixed with wholewheat pasta rings
- Lentil curry, lentil roast or lentil casserole
- Chicken and vegetable casserole or chicken tandoori served with plenty of cooked or salad vegetables, and baked potatoes, boiled potatoes, pasta, rice or bread
- Baked apple served with buttermilk
- Fruit and low-fat yoghurt
- Wholemeal bread pudding with mixed dried fruit, spice, low-fat milk and beaten egg

Simple Meals

- Poached egg and baked beans on toast
- Vegetables baked in the oven with an egg
- Scrambled egg or grilled fish on toast with sticks of celery or other salad vegetables
- Egg scrambled with a vegetable such as tomato, peas or sweetcorn
- Baked beans with cooked vegetables added and curry spices (optional) served with pitta bread
- Wholemeal or rye bread with a low-fat hard cheese and salad
- Lentils or beans in a vegetable soup with wholemeal bread
- Baked potatoes stuffed with yoghurt and lean ham or fish, or with a low-fat soft cheese or grated low-fat hard cheese
- Wholemeal sandwiches with a salad item and lean meat, grated low-fat hard cheese, fish, peanut butter, boiled egg, or a home-made lentil or bean spread. Suitable salad items include cress, tomato, cucumber, lettuce, chicory, sliced radish, onion, pepper or beansprouts. Banana and chopped nuts also makes a nice filling

Limiting Fat When Eating Out

This is where the problems can arise in cutting down on fat. You may find there are no satisfying low-fat foods to choose from when eating out, or that the lower-fat items such as roast meat or steak are too expensive. Another problem is that you cannot always assess how fatty, for example, a curry or a pasta dish will be. You may expect boiled potatoes and find they are swimming in butter or margarine.

Many of our study participants in fact ate less often in their work canteens or not at all in order to eat low-fat foods. But there are obvious dodges when eating out such as avoiding foods you know have been fried such as chips or fish in batter. Also avoid pastries, rich sauces, cream, dumplings, Yorkshire pudding, sausages and burgers if you can. As well as avoiding pastry steer clear of suet and sponge puddings, gâteaux and cheesecakes. As with achieving all the nutritional goals, if you eat out only very occasionally then choosing one of these higher-fat foods does not matter.

Other ways of reducing fat are to leave any butter on the table well alone – eat a bread roll without it. Similarly, forget about the cream or mayonnaise. Always try to choose vegetables without added fat and if you can fill up on bread and extra boiled or baked potatoes then you won't feel the need for a high-fat pudding. Fruit or a low-fat yoghurt make good choices. When choosing something like a ploughman's lunch or soup with bread, it may be worth asking for extra bread instead of your butter.

When regularly eating away from home your best solution may be to take with you home-made sandwiches with carefully chosen, interesting fillings. Fresh fruit is also convenient. When you are not having anything else sweet or high in fat you will need plenty of bread for your sandwiches in order to satisfy you.

Do not just accept that there are few low-fat choices – if you would like to see a better choice available make sure you let the manager know.

Children and the Fat in Their Diet

It is easy to bring children up eating a diet with a sensible level of fat in it. They will not miss fat in stews and casseroles or from chops, roast meats and gravies, if you have never used much fat in cooking. Avoiding chips most days won't be a hardship either if you have never cooked them at home. Many tasty dishes can be offered instead of burgers and sausages. If you do use them from time to time prick them well, grill them, drain off the fat and serve with other foods that are not high in fat. In-between-meals snacks can pose more of a problem when thinking about fat. But many foods are suitable. Suggestions are included in the section on between-meal snacks at the end of the chapter. But remember that some savoury sandwich fillings can be high in fat. Cheese and meat are good examples.

Ideally, all babies should be fed breast milk alone for the first 4–6 months of life. As it is not always possible to achieve 'the ideal' then it is perfectly safe for babies under 6 months who are not breastfed to be given a suitable modified milk formula. (Your Health Visitor will be able to advise you on this.) It is recommended by the DHSS that infants fed on infant formula milk continue on this until they are one year old.

After 6 months if you want to introduce ordinary cows' milk from a milk bottle or carton into your child's diet it is safe to do so. It is unwise to introduce skimmed milk at this stage.

Should you be giving your child vitamin drops, and if so which ones and how many? The DHSS advise that all infants be given 5 drops of A, D, C vitamin drops from the age of 1 month until the age of 2 years whether they are breast or bottle-fed.

Adjusting to Less Fat

• Don't suddenly cut down on the fat in your diet. It takes time to learn new enjoyable dishes that contain more carbohydrates that will make up the energy you will lose by not eating so much fat. This is particularly important for children. Cutting down too much on fat and too quickly could make them very hungry between meals, and some will turn to sweets, if only because children may not easily compensate for the loss of fat by eating more cereals and starchy foods. Less fat could therefore lead to weight loss and interfere with their growth (obviously this is less of a problem with overweight children).

● Make sure that you use your favourite flavourings and spices, vegetables and fruit, so that you don't miss the fat.

● Make a point of eating more potatoes, bread, pasta and rice so that you are not hungry.

● Avoiding high-fat convenience foods may mean doing more of your own cooking. Cook enough for two days or extra for your freezer.

● Don't ban all your favourite high-fat cheeses or meats, you might miss them and feel a lower-fat choice is a penance and not a pleasurable way of eating. Many of our participants said they could only continue with their improved diet if they could occasionally enjoy a high-fat cheese, cake or meat product.

● You may find you can enjoy a low-fat food taken with certain foods or drinks but not others – this was true for many who tried this healthier diet. For some, low-fat milk was acceptable in cooking and coffee, but not in tea.

● Gradually spread less fat on bread and leave it off altogether when appropriate.

● Gradually cut down the fat in your recipes as well as trying new low-fat recipes. Just making a gradual change will help you maintain your confidence in cooking.

Taste It, Don't Salt It! Eating Less Salt

What is Salt?

Salt is the common name for sodium chloride. There are numerous other salts such as potassium chloride, sodium bicarbonate or copper sulphate. When we say 'salt' in the nutritional context we are referring specifically to sodium chloride which is added to food or put on the roads in winter. Some records show that it is not just sodium chloride that should be reduced for good health, but other forms of sodium such as sodium bicarbonate in baking powder, or mono-sodium glutamate. However, most of the sodium in our diet does come from sodium chloride, so this is the main concern.

Over the last few hundred years we have taken to eating far more salt than we need. Salt is used to preserve food and also just for its taste (in many cases incidentally disguising the natural flavour of the food).

Most of the salt in our diet comes from processed foods and the majority is added to the food and is not naturally occurring. The salt you add to the food at home is obviously a source you can control to help reduce your salt intake. However, for most people this is the smaller part of the salt in their diet.

Sources of Salt in the Diet

33 per cent is added in cooking or at the table
33 per cent comes from cereals and bread
17 per cent comes from meat and meat products
17 per cent comes from all other foods

Some experts believe that even more of the salt we eat comes from the last three sources. One claims that as much as 88 per cent comes from sources over which the individual has no direct control.

How to Eat Less Salt

- Add only a little in cooking (if really necessary) and leave the salt off the table.
- Choose lower-salt foods to replace some of the salty foods you normally eat.

Lower-salt choice*	Higher-salt choice
Herbs, spices, lemon juice, garlic, home-made stocks, soups, vegetable water, vinegar, lemon juice	Stock cubes, meat and yeast extracts, pickles, tinned and packet soups, sauces, salt seasonings, sea salt, low-salt substitutes e.g. Prewetts
Oats, muesli, Puffed Wheat, Shredded Wheat	Cornflakes, Rice Krispies, Special K, Bran Flakes, All-Bran, Bran Buds (but check if salt is on the ingredients list)
Dried beans & lentils (you can make your own spreads with these)	Most cheeses
Lean fresh meat	Bacon, ham, salt beef, canned meat products, salami, sausages, burgers
Fresh and frozen fish	Smoked and tinned fish, shellfish, fish cakes, fish fingers
Fresh and frozen vegetables	Tinned vegetables
Sandwiches Pot of muesli with milk	Instant meals in pots
Nuts and raisins, fruit, raw vegetables	Crisps, salted nuts and biscuits
Unsalted butter and margarine	Butter and margarine

*less than 200mg of sodium per 100g of food

What Sort of Differences are There Between High-salt and Low-salt Choices?

Low-salt choice	% sodium*	High-salt choice	% sodium*
Frozen peas	0.002	Canned peas	0.2
Stewing steak (raw unsalted)	0.07	Corned beef	0.5 (some are higher)
Unsalted butter	0.06	Salted butter	0.9
Fresh haddock	0.1	Smoked haddock	1.2
Lentils – raw	0.04	Cheddar cheese	0.6
Lean pork	0.08	Streaky back bacon	1.5

*as salt is sodium chloride, the amount of sodium in the food indicates how much salt is present

What About Salt Substitutes?

A sensible aim should be to enjoy the natural flavour of food rather than crave for a salty taste. The situation is analogous to the use of artificial sweeteners. Taking salt substitutes doesn't really tackle the problem of wanting fewer salted foods. Most savoury, processed foods continue to contain salt which will be hard to avoid if you still have the taste for these salty foods. Some people find salt substitutes useful in weaning themselves off salt, and this should indeed be their main use. There are, however, drawbacks to salt substitutes: they are expensive (some are 27 times as expensive as salt, weight for weight); some substitutes still contain half salt; and there is still some doubt as to whether in the long run they are better than common salt – sodium chloride.

Sea salt, iodised salt, garlic salt and so on are not substitutes – they are all kinds of salt of which you should use less.

Shopping for Low-salt Foods

Most of the low-salt foods in the shops are basic commodities which have not had salt added during processing. Shellfish are an exception. Even fresh ones are high in salt but they really are not much of a problem – they are usually eaten in small amounts and can be boiled in unsalted water to reduce their salt content. The main problem to tackle is processed foods. You may find these have become an essential part of your life. You therefore need to choose sensibly and find ways of reducing salt that best suit your way of life. The following foods which are adequately low in salt should be found in most *large supermarkets*:

Oats, flour, pasta, rice
Pulses (dried)
Milk and eggs (in fact, these are naturally quite high in salt)
Fresh fish
Fresh meat – beef, pork, lamb, poultry, liver, kidney, rabbit
Fresh vegetables and fruit – most frozen vegetables (read the label)
Low-salt or low-sodium canned vegetables (may not be available)
Some tinned tomatoes do not contain salt
Fresh and frozen fruit or fruit juice
Canned or dried fruit
Unsalted, unsweetened muesli (may not be available)
Breakfast cereals without salt added
Breakfast cereals with salt low on the ingredients list
Unsalted nuts
Salt-free, polyunsaturated margarine (may not be available)
Unsalted butter
Cooking oil
Herbs and spices
Vinegar and lemon juice

To obtain the following low-salt foods you may have to visit a *large chemist or wholefood/health food shop*:

Muesli without added salt
Good variety of unsalted nuts and pulses
Good range of curry spices (or from an ethnic shop)
Good range of unrefined cereals and grains
Low-salt biscuits and crackers

Low-salt canned vegetables
Low-salt tomato or brown sauce
Reduced-salt yeast extract
Low-salt salad cream
Low-salt baked beans

If you are eating crisps, look out for salt-free crisps or the crisps with the little bag of salt which can be discarded.

Cakes, biscuits and bread from a local baker may be less salty than mass-produced supermarket breads.

Try not to put the following foods on your shopping list, or do so only occasionally:

Salted nuts, crisps and savoury biscuits
Bacon, ham, tinned meat, sausages, pâté, meat pie, salami, salted beef (silverside), salty yeast extracts, gravy powders
Smoked fish
Pickle
Bottled sauces
Packet and tinned soups

Cheese and tinned fish are also salty so try and eat a little less – choose fresh or frozen fish when you can. Cottage cheese is usually less salty than hard cheese, but you may need to consider how much you eat. If you eat more cottage cheese than hard at one time (because it is less dense) then it may not reduce your salt intake overall.

Reading the Labels

Reading the ingredients labels on foods is essential when trying to cut down on salt. Look out for the word salt or sodium on the list.

Tinned tomatoes are worth checking. Choose ones without salt. Breakfast cereals should also be checked if you want a change from unsalted muesli, Shredded Wheat or Puffed Wheat. Some have salt very low down the ingredient list so these are the next best choice. Also, check the labels of frozen vegetables and pasta.

You will also see on many packets of bread, biscuits and cakes that salt appears quite high up the ingredients list. For example, you may see on a packet of celery seed crackers that salt is higher up the list than celery seeds. Check pickles and sauces because these are high in salt too. Most cheeses will not have salt listed on the label even though they are high in salt. This is because salt is an essential part of their manufacture. Curd cheese and processed cheese are exceptions. These must state when salt is added.

What About Cost?

Eating a low-sodium diet costs less. Buying *fewer* processed foods and luxury foods such as salty snack biscuits and crisps (which are VAT rated), sauces and pickles saves money. But preparing more of your own foods can cost you more in fuel and time.

Buying special low-salt versions of products such as sauces and biscuits does cost more. Low-salt yeast extract costs nearly 60 per cent more than the full-salt variety in the same shop. You need to get your goal for salt into perspective. It is not necessary to rely on tinned vegetables regularly and why not cut down on the salty sauces, pickles and salted margarine rather than spend a lot of time and extra money buying the reduced-salt versions. After all, these are only a small part of the salt in your diet.

Buying special low-salt foods may be more important to you if you have high blood pressure in your family. You then need to work out the health benefit of buying these special low-salt products. In time they will probably become more widely available and no longer at premium prices.

Storing Your Low-salt Foods

Salt, like sugar, is used as a preservative. In spite of this, buying lower-salt foods should cause little problem with storage. Obviously a low-salt ham, bacon or salted fresh fish would cause problems to the manufacturer by having inadequate keeping qualities. You can simply avoid or choose less often those foods preserved with salt.

In the majority of cases salt is added for its flavour, and these lower-salt products will be no problem. Read the date mark if the product has one (tinned tomatoes probably do not) and follow the recommended storage conditions.

Plenty of low-salt foods make suitable reserves for when you cannot go out shopping. Examples are rice, pasta, flour, dried pulses, fruit and vegetables (frozen and tinned, and fresh with good keeping qualities) unsalted nuts and eggs. There is no reason, however, why you should not rely on cheese or tinned fish now and again.

Asking for Lower-Salt Foods

Reducing your salt intake is a hard goal to achieve if you lead a busy life and manufactured foods are a must. Bread, buns, crackers and crispbreads are all high in salt. These are foods which we are encouraged to eat more of. Making wholemeal bread is an excellent solution but not for everyone. Remember that you have the power to get foods you want stocked. If enough people write to the food manufacturer (chief executive or public relations department) and ask for a particular less salty food they will get it in time. Also, approach your supermarket manager about stocking less salty foods or have a word with your baker and ask if some of his bread is less salty than other types. Also, ask him if he thinks there is a demand for less salty bread and whether he might bake some.

Canteen food obviously varies from one canteen to another in its salt content, unless all the food is prepared from standard convenience foods. How much salt is added will probably depend on the cook's taste. The canteen won't know that you find the food too salty unless you say so. Point out that salt can be added to food by those who want it but not taken away once it's there.

Hints on Cutting Down on Salt at Home

● Careful shopping will prevent quite a lot of salt coming into your home.

● Leave the salt pot off the table; it is then far more effort to salt your food.

● If you must use a salt pot, choose one with one or a very few fine holes.

● For families with a baby, weaning can be a very useful time for all the family to reduce their salt intake. Young babies cannot tolerate much salt and they must not be given food with salt added or salty foods. This is therefore a marvellous opportunity to wean *yourself* off it. It is much easier to cook the same food for everyone. One of the Study's participants found their family's taste for salty food didn't return after weaning their baby.

Alternative Flavourings

● Food can taste bland when cutting down on salt so don't bore your taste buds – make good use of a variety of herbs, spices and flavourings. You will then be far less likely to miss the salt or to want to return to using it. Some of the ways herbs and spices can be used to flavour your foods are suggested on pages 155 to 157.

● Instead of the salt pot, put alternatives on the table, such as black, white or paprika pepper, cumin, mixed spice or nutmeg.

● Make your own mustard from mustard powder without adding salt, and mint sauce from fresh mint and vinegar.

Meat and Fish

● Don't salt your meat or fish before grilling or roasting. Use herbs and flavourings instead.

● When making stews, casseroles or gravy that need stock use the water saved after cooking vegetables. The other flavourings you use will compensate for the salt.

● By using fresh meat and fish rather than commercial fish

products and meat products you will not only be reducing your salt but probably your fat too.

Vegetables

• These have a wide variety of interesting flavours. Capitalise on this. Use plenty and choose a good mixture. The fresher the vegetable the better the flavour.
• When washing them never use salt.
• Try not to add salt or sodium bicarbonate in cooking. The latter reduces the nutritional value of the vegetables. It may be better to use just a pinch in cooking rather than end up adding a lot at the table.
• Liquidised vegetables can add flavour and texture to home-made soups and casseroles, helping to cut down on salt.
• When vegetables are steamed or baked there is no water to discard. Any salt you add therefore becomes more concentrated in your food. So if you cannot cut down altogether, use it very sparingly.

Wholegrain Rice and Pulses

• Without salt these cook much quicker and the skins do not harden.
• Use turmeric or cloves in the rice cooking-water for a change.
• Remember not to add a salty stock to your pulse dish – just use unsalted vegetable stock.

Baking

• There is no need to add a pinch of salt when baking buns, cakes, tea breads, biscuits, pastry etc.

Useful Herbs and Spices to Flavour Foods

Basil	Dried, for braised and stewed beef especially dishes containing tomato. Fresh, in salads

Bayleaf	For stocks and stews
Chives	Chopped finely and added to potatoes, tomatoes and salads
Coriander leaves	In salad; with lean chops
Garlic	Fresh only *not* garlic salt; crush and use with salads and meat, or to add to bean, lentil and pasta dishes. Goes well with tomato
Lemon	Lemon wedges with vegetables, salads, fish or tandoori chicken. Lemon rind and juice in chicken dishes and lentil, bean or fish curries
Mint	Lamb
Mixed herbs	Stews, stuffings and omelettes
Onion or shallot	Browned with beef or lamb or in a little oil with vegetables; baked with fish or grated in salad
Orange	Orange rind and juice in chicken dishes, beef stew or salad dressing
Parsley	Fish, chicken and vegetables
Rosemary	Lamb, chicken, fresh sardines and other oily fish; with white cabbage
Sage	Poultry, rabbit, chicken and turkey livers
Tarragon	Chicken and fish
Thyme	Stews; all poultry and pork dishes
Cayenne pepper	Vegetables and egg dishes
Cinnamon	With stewed fruit and in biscuits
Cloves	Pork and rice
Cumin	Sprinkled lightly on to vegetables, particularly courgettes and marrow
Ginger	Sprinkle on to pork or lamb chops before grilling or on to marrow
Mustard powder	Rub surface of meat e.g. kidney with dry mustard before cooking
Nutmeg	Grated over vegetables particularly cabbage, cauliflower or boiled potatoes
Peppercorns	Grind over most vegetables including

	lentil and bean dishes, also in beef or pasta dishes
Tandoori spice	To coat chicken
Turmeric	With wholegrain rice
Vinegar	Salads and fish

Hints on Cutting Down on Salt Away From Home

Try to avoid foods which you know are high in salt unless you only eat out rarely.

Don't add salt at the table – this you quite clearly have control over.

Take snacks with you which you know are fairly low in salt.

When there is a particular medical reason to cut down on salt you could ask your host not to add any salt when cooking. This is probably only realistic when you are staying for a few days.

Children and Salt

Children who are not introduced to salt from an early age are far less likely to acquire a taste for it. In an attempt to keep children away from sweets and sugary foods (for the benefit of their teeth) savoury foods are often encouraged. This can cause the development of a 'salty tooth'. Don't feel that you cannot win, just try and adopt a sensible approach. Many of the highly-processed meat products that appeal to children such as burgers, sausages or pies are also high in fat. You therefore have two reasons for not having them every day. Why not take the attitude, as with sweet foods, that the high-salt foods are not everyday foods – they are occasional foods.

Try to get your children into the habit of spending weekly pocket money on non-food items or fruit. When you want to bring a little surprise home, think of something like a pen, a comic, a children's magazine, a colouring book or a notepad instead.

Even if you find it difficult to curb the habit of adding salt to your food when cooking or adding it at the table – do it for your children. If Dad sprinkles his food liberally with salt you can't be surprised if the children will want to copy. You can only get away for just so long with pretending to sprinkle it on their plates! Also, don't get into the habit of putting lots of sauces on the table. Your children will never learn the natural flavour of food this way.

When they are away from home it is inevitable that they will be offered salty food. To some extent you may be able to educate your close friends and relatives to use less salt. You can also try and encourage your children not to add salt themselves when they go out. They probably will not want to if you don't use much at home.

Adapting to Less Salt

Don't feel you have got to make these changes overnight. Gradually put less salt in the food. Other family members adjust more easily this way too. Gradually let the salty, processed foods get into your shopping basket less often. Balance a salty choice such as ham, smoked fish or quiche with a low-salt choice such as fresh vegetables or pasta and fresh fruit to follow.

Always taste food before adding salt – don't just add it through habit.

Try to choose your favourite flavoured foods and vegetables more often to compensate for some of the highly-flavoured salty foods.

Think about hidden sources of salt in your food. Be extra careful not to add salt to a dish if you are also adding, for example, a low-calorie salad cream, tinned fish, grated cheese or Worcester sauce. These already have salt added. A *little* salt added when cooking a home-made dish is still likely to be far less salty than a bought, manufactured version. Let visitors adapt to your lower-salt cooking. You can always let them add salt – even though this may not be a habit you want young children to follow.

Dying for a Drink: Drink Less Alcohol

What is Alcohol?

Alcohol is produced by fermenting foods. It is the highest source of energy after fat – more fattening than sugar, other carbohydrates or protein. It is basically a poison to the body, particularly when more is consumed at one time than the body can cope with.

Women cannot usually tolerate as much alcohol as can men because their liver seems to fare less well when it comes to detoxifying the alcohol. The alcohol goals for this Study were based on a certain percentage of energy coming from alcohol. As women need less energy, the sex difference is allowed for. On the whole, this goal was the easiest to achieve (along with cutting down on sugar) for our Study participants. Many took very little alcohol anyway but some found the goal hard to achieve in hot weather when their desire for beer increased. One of our study weeks was in the summer when the weather was very hot.

Eating a healthy diet with adequate fibre and not too much sugar and fat should make you feel fitter and more able to tackle life. Try and create a way of life that suits you. You should then feel less need to drink more than the healthy goal that was set. This goal enables you safely to enjoy daily about two of the following drinks for women and between two and three for men (these are all based on pub measures):

  one glass of wine
  half a pint of beer or lager
  one measure of spirits
  one glass of sherry or Martini.

This allowance is plenty to accomodate most people's normal, social drinking.

A Sensible Attitude to Alcohol

Although we are all encouraged to cut down on alcohol, there is no evidence that light drinkers (drinking less than the limit above) are less healthy than those who abstain. After all, non-drinkers may have a compensatory higher intake of sugar and fat. On the contrary, research suggests that those who drink a little alcohol might have *fewer* heart attacks than those who don't drink at all.

It is worth remembering that alcohol is very fattening. Most people take alcoholic drinks for reasons other than to satisfy their hunger or thirst and they can end up taking a lot of surplus calories. Alcohol also stimulates the appetite so beware if excess weight is your problem!

Alcohol can be a trouble-maker: it is expensive so before buying make sure you can afford the other foods you need to stay healthy as well as to pay for your non-food bills; it can be the start of many rows and fights; it causes accidents – especially road accidents; and it changes personalities.

Couples who are thinking of starting a family should keep their alcohol intake very low or preferably abstain altogether for the three months before conception and a woman should stay off alcohol all during pregnancy. Even very small intakes of alcohol have been found adversely to affect the unborn baby.

It is also advisable when taking certain drugs not to drink at all. Ask your doctor about this.

How to Cut Down on Alcohol

● Start to dissociate drinking alcohol from certain occasions. Build other pleasures into the occasions on which you used to drink alcohol. Let these pleasures be totally removed from extra food. Some good ideas are: reading the weekend paper, having a bubble bath, playing a game, eating your meal outdoors, playing with your children, making love – whatever you enjoy.
● Make your drinks smaller – buy a spirit measure for home. Order halves and singles when you are out.

● As with children who are cutting down on sweets, put the money you save on alcohol each week into a jar. Decide what good use you will put it to and look forward to that thing. It is always difficult giving up a pleasure but it is far easier if you can give yourself another 'present' to look forward to.

● Alternate alcoholic drinks with non-alcoholic drinks.

● At a meal have two glasses – one for water and one for your alcoholic drink. Leave the alcoholic drink until the end of the meal when it cannot be topped up.

● Dilute wine with sparkling mineral water. This is very refreshing in the summer, especially with white wine.

● Dilute beer by making a shandy.

● Non-alcoholic beers are now available. See if these could become an adequate substitute for you.

● If you do drink heavily spend some time deciding why. If necessary seek professional help on this. Start, perhaps, by seeing your doctor or going to a meeting of a local self-help group. If your drinking is nothing but habit then the hints above should help you begin to learn new ones. Your drinking may, of course, go much deeper. If this is the case for you it is probably time you started to tackle the underlying causes. No situation is totally unchangeable – even if it just means gradually changing the way you view it. Heavy drinking will not solve that underlying problem – it usually needs professional help.

The New Way of Eating

Now that we have looked at achieving the main goals individually you may now be wondering what there is left to eat! As we mentioned before, the secret of success is *not* to look for 'perfect' foods; it is more a matter of making a little progress here and there wherever you can. The beauty of the whole thing is that once you have made a start things get easier all the time. Once you cut down on sugar you start to taste the natural sweetness of things (especially fruit and vegetables) and even savoury foods taste better. If you then reduce the amount of salt you take even foods containing no added salt taste quite pleasantly salty from their own natural salts.

Slowly, your palate becomes re-educated and eating takes on a new pleasure. This can be more than doubled if you also stop smoking. Many people report that after stopping smoking they can taste and enjoy foods they had forgotten about long ago. Nicotine stifles the taste-buds and one's sense of smell and this could be a reason for so many people needing such sweet and salty foods if they are to taste them at all. Some ex-smokers say it is like a blind man receiving his sight back – so wonderful is it to be free from the taste-dulling experiences of nicotine.

But however you decide to eat you will have to buy the right foods and have good, wholesome food at hand for when you want it. Let's start off, therefore, by looking at what sorts of things you should have at home if you are to eat more healthily.

Foods to Store at Home

Wholemeal bread
Wholewheat pasta
Wholegrain rice
100% wholewheat flour
Wholewheat or wholerye crispbreads
Wholewheat biscuits
Wholegrain cereals
Oats, wheat, barley, millet or rye flakes
Wholemeal scones, fruit bread or buns
Tinned fish
Fresh, white or oily fish, poultry or fresh, lean meat
Eggs
Skimmed or semi-skimmed milk

Low-fat hard and soft cheeses
Low-fat sugar-free yoghurt
Split peas, chick peas
One or more kinds of dried beans and lentils
Tinned beans
Tinned vegetables
Fruit tinned in natural juice
Frozen fruits and vegetables
Dried fruits
Unsalted nuts
Caraway, sunflower, sesame and pumpkin seeds
Unsweetened pickles
Vinegar
Mustard
Herbs

Pepper and other spices, garlic

Oil, margarine

Low-calorie or diabetic fruit squash

Store some of the following if you have a freezer:
home-made low-fat casseroles: meat, bean or lentil
a nut roast
fish pie with potato topping
fruit crumble
wholemeal scones
cooked beans ready to use.

Having got all your healthy foods together you may well need to start planning your eating rather differently. Here are a few ideas for meals.

Quick Breakfast Ideas
● Large helping of wholegrain cereal with low-fat milk – add dried fruit or sliced fresh fruit on top for a change
● Wholemeal toast with peanut butter or low-fat soft cheese or curd cheese (medium-fat);
● Muesli (with no sugar added) with natural yoghurt with grated apple or sliced banana. This is nice soaked overnight and delicious with red fruit or blackcurrants when in season. Also good as a dessert;
● Warmed wholemeal bread – a hunk, a roll, or part of a brown French stick, thinly spread with margarine if desired, with a natural low-fat yoghurt, a banana;
● Rye bread with a low-fat hard cheese and small glass of unsweetened fruit juice;
● Stewed fruit (no added sugar) or dried fruit compôte topped with natural yoghurt and then a flaked cereal – rye, barley or wheat.

Cooked or Leisurely Breakfasts
● Baked beans on toast;
● Poached egg on toast;
● Boiled egg, wholemeal toast with margarine and a little marmalade;

● Fish fingers and grilled tomatoes with a wholemeal bread roll;

● Unsweetened fruit juice, large helping of porridge with low-fat milk. Add dried fruit during cooking for a change;

● Half a grapefruit, scrambled egg (just egg and low-fat milk in a non-stick pan) on a wholemeal bap;

● Wholemeal bread dipped in beaten egg, seasoned with pepper or nutmeg. Both sides cooked in a lightly greased non-stick pan;

● Vary your choice – not an egg every day!

Main Meal Ideas

● Shepherd's pie. Remember to drain off the fat from the mince. Add extra vegetables to the mince mixture. Top with a thick layer of low-fat mashed potato. Brown rice pudding – made with skimmed milk and dried fruit for sweetening;

● Bean shepherd's pie: pre-cooked or canned beans mixed with frozen mixed vegetables and fresh or tinned tomatoes, herbs plus a little water with a topping of plenty of low-fat mashed potato. Banana split – slice in two and fill with natural yoghurt, and a spoonful of crunchy cereal or nuts;

● Liver, bacon and vegetable casserole. Use back bacon and brown the liver with the bacon and onions if used. Serve with baked potatoes or wholegrain rice and an extra vegetable. Baked apple stuffed with dried fruit and mixed spice;

● Nut roast. Make like a meat loaf, replacing meat with finely chopped nuts (see recipe on page 202). Serve with fresh or tinned tomatoes and baked potatoes and a mixed green salad;

● Lentil curry with wholegrain rice and a cucumber and yoghurt raita (chopped cucumber and yoghurt with mint and minced garlic optional);

● Kidney and bean casserole (see recipe, page 199) – with wholegrain rice and cauliflower or cabbage;

● Grilled, small, lean pork chops – spoonful of stewed apple, with carrots and spring greens, potatoes boiled in their jackets. Fruit – tinned in natural juice topped with yoghurt;

● Chicken and vegetable casserole (remove skin from chicken) with wholegrain rice and vegetables baked in the oven. Baked dried fruit compôte with chopped nuts on top;

● Rabbit and vegetable casserole served with mixed mashed potato and swede (using low-fat milk and pepper – the potato skins can be mashed too). Wholemeal bread pudding;

● Grilled grapefruit. (Add a teaspoon of sherry or crème de menthe as a treat.) Baked herrings or mackerel. Casserole of sliced potato and onion with a little low-fat milk seasoned with herbs and pepper;

● White fish baked with onions, tomatoes, pepper and garlic (optional), parsley or tarragon. With baked potatoes and fresh or frozen green beans;

● Wholewheat spaghetti bolognese. Halve the mince in ordinary recipes and supplement with tinned or pre-cooked beans. After browning the mince with vegetables, discard fat from the meat. Serve with mixed salad tossed in a lemon and oil dressing (2 parts lemon, 1 part oil) and wholemeal bread;

● Wholewheat lasagne – make a skimmed milk and cornflower sauce using just a little strongly flavoured cheese. Lentils can be used to replace mince. Serve with Chinese leaf and orange salad;

● Cauliflower cheese – sauce made as for lasagne. Serve with huge hunk of wholemeal bread or baked potato. Wholemeal scone (see recipe page 201);

● Beef and bean casserole – your usual beef and vegetable casserole recipe, reduce the meat and add pre-cooked beans (any kind) and no added fat or oil. Baked spiced banana;

● Grilled sardines or mackerel rubbed with garlic and rosemary. New potatoes in their jackets; tomato and beansprout salad. Apple;

● Spanish omelette, containing peas, potato, pepper, mushrooms (optional). Cook in a greased non-stick pan. Serve with broccoli or spinach and crusty wholemeal French stick. Fruit salad, using unsweetened fruit;

● Roast chicken, pork or beef (remove skin and fat) – roast potatoes (parboil then lightly brush potato with oil before browning off in the oven). Gravy from the vegetable stock. Sprouts and braised leeks. Gooseberry and strawberry wholemeal crumble (or other fruit in season). See recipe, page 202;

● Chicken or turkey and nut risotto – cook in a non-stick pan with just a little oil; add onions, peas, corn, tomato, celery or mushrooms as available. Dried fruit compôte with yoghurt.

Simpler Meals

● Scrambled egg with sweetcorn on wholemeal bread bap. Sticks of celery and fresh tomato (when in season);

● Curried beans – add curry powder and cooked or tinned vegetables to baked beans. Add a little water if required. Or use other tinned beans plus tomato purée and a little more water. Wholemeal pitta bread. Crisp lettuce or Chinese leaf with chopped chives and onions;

● Grilled fish fingers, frozen peas, boiled potatoes or wholemeal toast;

● Grilled pilchards or sardines – for a change, add finely chopped onion, celery and pepper to the fish and mash. Wholemeal toast and watercress;

● Home-made lentil soup (pasta can be added). Wholemeal or granary bread (for a change). Apple or orange;

● Grated cheese grilled on toast or on French stick sliced open, with tomatoes on top. Cucumber and tomato salad;

● Tuna fish and wholemeal pasta – as shells or rings. Brown onion or pepper in little of fish oil. Mix in fish, peas, cooked pasta, any other cooked vegetables or corn. Green salad or cabbage;

● Salad of lean, cooked meat or mixed unsalted nuts. Home-made coleslaw with yoghurt dressing. Potato salad (see recipe on page 198), shredded lettuce, wholemeal bread;

● Home-made leek and potato soup. Stuffed pitta bread – shredded mixed vegetables tossed with prawns, lemon juice and little yoghurt (plus low-calorie salad cream – optional). Chopped nuts or cooked chicken can replace prawns;

● Egg baked in the oven on a nest of frozen, mixed veget-

ables, plus tomato juice, served with baked potato or whole-wheat pasta;
● Ploughman's lunch consisting of low-fat soft cheese, Edam or other reduced-fat hard cheese or small portion (up to 45g) of your favourite cheese. Large helping wholemeal bread, salad in season, pickled onion or gherkin. Fruit jelly made with gelatine, unsweetened fruit juice and fruit (no jelly cubes).

Between-meals Snacks

This is where many of the Study participants had difficulty. They felt hungry as a result of having less sugar and fat at meals and ran out of ideas for suitable in-between-meals snacks.

It is relatively easy to make tasty meals which have a controlled level of fat, sugar and salt. Finding convenient snacks for between meals is not so easy. Put your efforts into your meals and then make the best choice you can if you are hungry between meals. Overall your efforts should balance out.

Try to fill up on potatoes, bread and other starchy foods at meals, but here are some suitable snack ideas if you do feel hungry . . . and you probably will over the first few weeks until you get used to eating much larger, bulkier meals.

● Fresh fruit – vary your choice
● Wholemeal sandwiches with salad, banana or peanut butter fillings
● Wholemeal bread, toast or crispbread spread with a thin layer of polyunsaturated margarine or low-fat spread
● Mixed raw vegetables in finger-sized pieces
● Home-made, wholemeal bread or rolls, fruit soda bread, fruit muffins, teabread, scones or griddle cakes
● Bought wholemeal scones or wholemeal currant buns or muesli buns
● Dried fruits and unsalted nuts
● Wholegrain cereal with low-fat milk

Take a snack with you when you go out if you are likely to need one. Wrap it with some cling film or put it in a plastic bag.

Packed Meals
(to take to school, work or for outings)

Wedge of cheese or small carton of cottage cheese
Large hunk of wholemeal bread
Stick of celery, tomato or carrot
Water or soup in a flask

Liver sausage and cucumber sandwich
Grated cheese and piccalilli sandwich
Currant bun
Pear
Diluted natural fruit juice

Home-made lentil soup in a flask
Large hunk of granary bread or two wholemeal baps
Stick of celery
Yoghurt

Wholemeal muffins with egg, tomato and cress filling
Digestive biscuit
Banana

Cheese scones – home-made and wholemeal
Celery, nuts and raisins
Banana sandwich
Diluted fruit juice

Wholegrain pasta or rice salad with chopped ham, flaked tuna fish, nuts or cooked, dried beans and peas, sweetcorn, diced pepper, celery or green beans and a low-fat dressing. Put in a sealed container.
Apple
Handful of crunchy cereal

Slice of cheese flan (try wholemeal flour pastry)
Carton of crunchy salad
Wholemeal bread, thinly spread with margarine
Fresh fruit

Small pizza (try wholemeal base)
Carton of mixed salad
Wholemeal scone
Apple

Pitta bread stuffed with mixed grated vegetable (try carrot, cabbage, onion, bean-sprouts, apple)
Peanuts or mixed peanuts and sunflower seeds in a carton
Slice of tea bread or fruit loaf

Chicken thigh or drumstick

Carton of home-made
potato salad with
yoghurt dressing
Tomato
Large slice of crusty brown
French bread
Handful of 'tropical mix' or
dried fruit

Peanut butter sandwich
Lentil paste sandwich (see
sandwich fillings)
Wholemeal fruit crumble
put in a carton

Milk or milk shake
Hot drink in flask
Slice of home-made meat
or nut loaf
Coleslaw in container
(make your own to last
several days)
Sesame seed roll
Scotch pancake or griddle
cake
Orange

Sandwich Fillings

Vary the choice because some are high in salt and others high
in fat. Sandwiches, except those with wet fillings, can be made
in bulk and frozen.

Cheese. Grated or sliced, or curd cheese – with tomato,
low-sugar pickle, onion, grated apple or carrot; flavoured
cottage cheese

Meat. Sliced ham, corned beef, tongue, haslet, chicken – with
pickle, mustard, shredded lettuce, cucumber, tomato. Instead
of margarine try a low-calorie salad cream some days.

Fish. Tuna, sardines, pilchards or mackerel (drained of oil),
prawns – with lemon juice or low-calorie salad cream, plus
shredded lettuce, chopped onion or pepper, tomato or
cucumber

Nuts/Beans. Mashed banana with peanut butter or chopped
nuts, bean or lentil paste (beans or lentils boiled or baked to
a thick paste with stock, onions, other vegetables and
flavourings see pages 155 to 157.

More Vegetables and Fruit Ideas to Pack

- Add vegetables to sandwich fillings where possible.
- Wrap separate items, e.g. celery, raw carrot, tomato,

fennel, Cos lettuce or Chinese leaf, cucumber in cling film. Fresh fruit, dried fruits.

● Carton salads. Try combinations of shredded red and green cabbage, celery, carrot, apple, Chinese leaf, fennel, cauliflower, sprouts, diced pepper, cooked peas, green beans, nuts, dried fruit, seeds (sunflower, sesame) with a dressing of vinegar, orange or lemon juice, yoghurt, oil or low-calorie salad cream. Potato salad.

● Wholemeal fruit crumble, tinned fruit in natural juice, stewed fruit – in sealed container.

Encouraging Others to Eat Healthily

Why Bother?

First you need to think about whether you want to encourage others to eat healthily and why. There are a number of reasons to influence others to eat more healthily.

Healthy eating in a family setting means at least some involvement by all the family members and this can be beneficial to the family as a whole. It gets them talking to each other and thinking about their health both individually and as a unit. Such discussions teach children that parents have a responsibility to guard their children's health, both now and for the future.

You may be concerned that all your family members benefit from a healthier diet and not just yourself as a parent.

You may already have strong medical reasons to change your own or your family's eating habits, such as a history of heart disease, overweight members in the household, diabetes or a bowel disorder. If altering the way you eat makes sense for you on these grounds, it certainly does so for your children, if only because the sooner you start them off on the right path the less likely they are to suffer from the family's pre-disposition to the particular disease or ailment.

You may be concerned about your friends' or relatives' health and want to share both your knowledge and the pleasure you get from eating more healthily.

You may want to influence your friends and relatives so it is easier for you to eat more healthily when you visit them or they visit you.

Influencing your work's canteen, school meals service, local café, pub, restaurant or take-away, may help both you and total strangers to eat more healthily.

Lastly, there is the feeling we all have that if we are enjoying something we want to share it with others.

How can you do it?

Before expecting others to change their attitudes, think about why you wanted to eat healthier food and what influenced you. Think about what is in it for those you want to influence. This should help you in your efforts to involve others. The tactics you adopt and compromises you exercise may be different depending on who you want to influence and why.

Food is a very emotive and sometimes powerful issue – more so in some families than others. Food is used as an expression of care or love. For example 'I have cooked (or bought) this because John (or Mary) is ill/upset/having a difficult time', 'My mother-in-law is coming to stay, I must serve her favourite cake and biscuits.' Serving your guests their favourite foods or companies providing a special dining room for their top staff are other examples of caring through food. Most people gain considerable security from their food and are at least temporarily anxious at the thought of having to change anything about it. They see it as a part of their 'normal' and accepted lifestyle and most need to be given very good reasons for making changes at all. Here are a few tips to bear in mind.

When making changes that involve others, try not to undermine the feelings of security they obtain from eating. For example, don't change most of your spouse's or family's favourite foods all at once. If wholemeal rice or pasta is not popular, alternate it with the old food habits. Also, there are many ways of expressing your care for others without regularly doling out excessive amounts of sugar, fat, salt or alcohol. Coming home on time, doing the washing up or ironing or saying you are sorry might go down just as well or even better than a box of chocolates. Serving foods to please your friends or relatives could mean remembering they like fresh pineapple, shrimps or fresh Brussels sprouts. The fact that they also love a good cheese board or cream cakes which you don't normally serve doesn't prove that you don't care. Serving others sensibly chosen foods most of the time means that you *do* care. Their health is important to you – that *is* caring. Unfortunately, once you step out of the confines of your immediate family such care, however genuine, can be misunderstood and even be seen as 'busy-bodying' or unwanted interference. Go gently and be tactful. Remember that your motivations for changing to a healthier diet might not have any relevance to them.

Don't be a bore about food. A casual attitude to healthy eating with no radical changes is a sensible approach.

Expect some of your attitudes about food to rub off on others, but not all.

Help others to understand the benefits of healthy eating, but don't force it down their throats. It helps if people know the reasons why you are making changes, but don't necessarily expect them to accept your reasons as being good enough for them.

Decide on your level of compromise with others, based on why you want to make changes. A strong medical reason always makes things simpler.

Adopt some obvious changes and other more subtle, less obvious ones. Give way on some habits that are important to your family and friends. For example, you may want to change to brown rice, to stop having puddings during the week and have chips once a week instead of three or more times. Less obvious changes might be to buy a different margarine – a low-fat variety or one high in polyunsaturates; to change your milk order to semi-skimmed and to stop using fat in cooking. Some members of the family may hunger for burgers and sausages. If this is the case, serve these some days – grill them and serve vegetables without fat added.

The first changes to make in your household should be the ones most members of the family will accept, then introduce new habits that seem very important to *you* (you will then be more able to accept the consequences for these).

Don't give up after one attempt with a new food. Because of

the security people gain from familiar foods, the first time something new is introduced, it might be a shock. Like yourself, others get used to new foods and habits and then don't want to return to the old ones. Many people, once they have given up sugar in tea and coffee cannot drink it if it is sweetened and this goes for other things including salty or fatty foods.

Rows or 'taking a stand' over new eating habits are unlikely to achieve your aims. The harder you push, the harder others will retaliate. Gentle persuasion with no rigid rules is the answer. Find the best compromise. In most families likes and dislikes can often be easily catered for. For example, if one member of a family dislikes fish, he or she could be given a portion of something left over from the previous day. Other members of the family can then enjoy fish sometimes. Alternatively, a certain dish can be eaten when a member of the family, who dislikes that dish, is eating elsewhere. Obviously, meals liked by all members of the family are eaten more often than those which are popular with only one or a few. The same kind of compromise should be exercised when introducing healthy eating. It's a matter of everyone bending a little and the cook using some common sense!

Don't forget that if members of the family are eating some meals outside this can be an opportunity for them to eat their old, unhealthy favourites.

Don't be afraid of occasionally taking a stand if members of your household are old enough to buy their own foods. Don't feel guilty if you have not bought the unnecessary foods such as fancy cakes, biscuits or bottled sauces. With younger members of the household, if they question your changes, explain why you have made them.

Make the changes colourful and interesting. If you know, for example, that mushrooms are popular, use them in your new dish.

On a very practical level, remember to encourage more of the starchy foods or the hunger from eating less sugar and fat will discourage others from accepting the changes because they will feel hungry so much of the time – as many of our participants did.

Healthy Food in a Hurry

Many of the participants in our study felt they had spent longer preparing their food when eating more healthily. A few, however, recorded that it had taken less time. It is not surprising that you might need more time. Avoiding fat, sugar and salt and guaranteeing that a wholegrain cereal is used unfortunately often means preparing your own. But it is less of a problem than it at first appears. As healthy eating becomes a way of life new habits quickly become automatic and probably involve only a little extra time.

When you are in a hurry it may be a matter of making the best of convenience foods. Here are some tips:

- The freezer can be very useful – if you have one, use it. Cook large batches and freeze them in one meal or as single snack-sized portions for other days. This reduces your cooking and washing-up time.
- Plan ahead with your catering so that you can take deadlines into your stride. For example, slice enough onions for two days if you know they will be needed for tomorrow as well. Clean two days' worth of carrots at a time, store them, once cleaned, in a plastic bag in the fridge. Think on your way home what you need to do to prepare the meal so you can proceed without delay.
- Bread and pasta dishes are quick but with potatoes and wholegrain rice you can cook double the quantity the day before. Pre-cooked rice can be used in a risotto or rice salad, or for stuffing vegetables. Potatoes can be mashed or sliced and be heated as a potato topping, or used for a potato salad or added to a quickly prepared Spanish omelette.
- Think ahead with beans – soak overnight. They can also be cooked the previous evening (after soaking all day) and then just added to vegetables the next day.
- Buy a chicken or joint larger than you need for one meal and store the leftover meat in a fridge. Use the cold meat for a casserole, risotto or pasta dish the following day.
- When making a quick curry with cooked meat, lentils and vegetables try wholemeal pitta bread as an accompaniment if you have insufficient time to cook wholegrain rice.

● One-pot meals can save time as there is less washing up to do.

● Tinned fish, tinned beef or ham and eggs can be handy for quick meals from time to time.

Balancing the Cost

The cost of altering the fibre, sugar, fat, salt and alcohol content of your diet has been considered separately under each section but what will the cost of altering the way you eat mean overall?

We costed out one weekday's food from the 'before' and 'after' diaries of one of our participants. The first diary showed what she was spending on food normally and the second when she was eating more or less according to our guidelines. In fact, her energy intake was lower in the second diary (as was the case with most of our participants) even though there did not seem to be less food. We therefore added extra snacks to the second diary to make a fair comparison. Obviously it's cheaper if you are eating less.

Diary 1

Breakfast	2 slices white bread spread with butter and marmalade
	cup of coffee with a dash of whole milk and 2 teaspoons of sugar
Midday	A third of a 340g (12 oz) quiche
	large helping of Brussels sprouts
	one small carton of cheesecake
Evening	250g (9oz) roast chicken leg
	frozen peas
	white sauce made from whole milk and margarine
	1 wholemeal bap
	apple
	coffee with whole milk and 2 teaspoons of sugar

Snacks	2 small glasses of fresh orange juice
	1 chocolate digestive biscuit
	1 cup of tea with whole milk

Diary 2

Breakfast	3 Weetabix with semi-skimmed milk
	1 slice of wholemeal bread, thinly spread with low-fat spread
	coffee with a dash of semi-skimmed milk

| Midday | 3 slices of wholemeal bread, thinly spread with low-fat spread, 2 slices, 56g (2oz), lean boiled ham, mixed salad of lettuce, tomato and cucumber, a banana with one carton of natural low-fat yoghurt |

Evening	Wholewheat lasagne with a lentil, tomato, onion and green pepper sauce cooked in a teaspoon of oil
	jacket potato
	apple
	tea with a dash of semi-skimmed milk

Snacks	Wholemeal spiced fruit bun, thinly spread with low-fat spread
	30g (1oz) salted nuts and raisins
	cup of coffee with a dash of semi-skimmed milk

All the food for both the first and the second diaries was priced in a large supermarket, based on average packet sizes. *The old way of eating in Diary 1 was calculated to be 14.5 per cent more expensive than the new way of eating in Diary 2. Both menus provided about the same energy value of 2000 calories. For many people the new way of eating can actually save money.* The participants in the Study on the whole felt that they were spending no more on food when eating more healthily. Although a few felt they were spending more, this was balanced by others who thought it was cheaper. Many of the participants were already buying the more expensive wholegrain products so there was little extra to pay for these when changing to the new diet. Also, the majority of participants did not appear to be wasting any money overeating in the first or second diaries. Those in our study who found the new way of eating cheaper were avoiding unnecessary VAT-rated items and were exploring ways with beans and lentils. Those participants who commented the new way was dearer were replacing cheese and cheaper convenience foods with lean meat. With a little thought and planning a way can usually be found to eat healthily without increasing the cost.

The Balance

Money-savers	Extra expenses
Less meat – replacing or supplementing with beans or lentils some days	Changing from fatty and salty meat products to leaner meat and fish
Less cheese	Some low-fat, hard cheeses, stronger-flavoured cheeses
Fewer sweets and chocolates and other VAT-rated foods	More vegetables and fruits
Fewer cakes and biscuits and replacing fancy ones with simpler breads, buns and biscuits	Fruits in natural juice rather than syrup
Fewer manufactured puddings and desserts	More bread, rice, pasta, flour and cereals
Low-fat milk to replace whole milk and less cream	Wholegrain products instead of fibre-depleted processed ones
Less sugar and 'visible' fats – margarine, butter, suet etc	More fuel for cooking some of the main dishes
Generally buying simpler and less processed foods	

Making Cost Savings on Your Food

- Use the most economical source for your shopping – don't forget to add in your bus fares, petrol or taxi when working out costs. Large supermarkets with a reputation for freshness are probably the cheapest except for fresh vegetables, fruits and nuts. Try to use one of the following for these; market stalls with a good reputation, farm shops, local small-holdings selling by the roadside, greengrocers with a fast turnover and reasonable price, or your own allotment or vegetable patch. Explore whether there is a health-food co-operative in your area. A local vegetarian group or society will know. You can make great savings buying from such an outlet.
- Buy vegetables and fruits when they are in season, and cook or serve them in different ways. When tomatoes are in season citrus fruits are often expensive. When tomatoes become a luxury the reverse is true. They are both good sources of Vitamin C so buying whichever is in season makes good economic sense.

Fresh fruit and vegetables are usually the cheapest but in late spring frozen vegetables may be useful.

- Always read the weights on packaged foods so you know how much you are getting for the price – carry a pocket calculator with you if necessary. Buy a larger packet if it is economical but check you will eat it before the 'best before' date.
- Beware of fancy packaging – there is no point paying for upmarket paper or plastic when you have gone to buy food.
- Make use of special offers but weigh up the costs – will the food be eaten before it goes off? A freezer can be useful for storing foods which are reduced for quick sale but remember to eat it all on the day you unfreeze it. Introductory offers can be an excellent buy. It may be worthwhile stocking up, for example, on tinned fruit in natural juice or wholegrain rice but do remember their storage lives.
- Write a shopping list. This not only helps when making changes to the products you buy but also keeps down the cost. It ensures that you buy only what you need – that

nothing is wasted and that no extra shopping trips are required. All of these trips cost money you need not spend.
● Check date stamping carefully. Buy the one with the latest date. This reduces the likelihood of having to throw out food.
● If you are overweight think of all the money you have wasted buying fat and sugar you didn't need – you will soon have pounds in your pocket instead of on you!
● Remember that sweets, confectionery, chocolate, biscuits, crisps and savoury snacks as well as soft drinks are VAT-rated. You are therefore paying more for these foods. Buying less will make valuable savings.
● Taking a packed meal to work or school may save money provided there is time available for its preparation.

Can Social Eating be Healthy Eating?

Social eating can be fitted in with healthy eating although it can be difficult if you often eat out. However, healthy eating need not jeopardise a happy social life.

Entertaining at Home

When you are entertaining take the attitude 'When in Rome do as the Romans do'. Let your visitors get used to your way of eating. There is no need to ban butter, cream, salty foods, sweet desserts, alcohol or crusty white French bread. You may feel this is an occasion to celebrate or you may like something different for a change. Don't go overboard, however. Make sure there is a choice for your visitors to eat healthily if they want to. Offer two puddings for example, something like a fruit trifle balanced by an unsweetened fruit salad. Don't automatically butter bread for a starter or add butter to potatoes. Let your visitors have a choice. After all, they may eat out a lot.

There is no need to be a martyr either. This draws attention to yourself. If you want to keep an eye on your fat, salt and sugar, plan your meals so that it is easy for you. Have more or less the same on your plate but leave off the sauce, butter, salt, cream or ice cream. There are plenty of subtle ways of watching your diet.

Eating Out with Others

This may pose more problems than entertaining at home.

If you eat out regularly make the best choice you can. Introducing new healthy ideas to your friends when you entertain should gradually start to influence them. It will then become easier when you visit them. Eating out in restaurants with friends or business associates can be a problem. Take the initiative and recommend a place that you know serves healthy foods.

Many of our Study participants found it so difficult to eat healthily in their works' canteens that they took packed meals. You may find this excludes you from valuable social contact. Eating in the canteen on alternate days could be a solution.

It is often true that like-minded people stick together. You may find that your friends would like to eat healthier foods when you eat with each other – but it may just need you to take the lead.

Try not to make a fuss about your food – on the other hand don't use social eating as an excuse not to eat well. Follow your convictions and ask for wholemeal bread or boiled potatoes or bread in place of chips.

It can often be easier than you think to eat healthily at a 'finger buffet'. Steer clear of the vol-au-vents, sausage rolls, sausages and crisps. Head for the sandwiches, bread rolls and any vegetable or salad items (which are thankfully becoming more commonplace).

Eating Out in General

Everyone eats at least some food prepared – and ready-to-eat – outside their homes at some time. Just how often they eat out and why varies but for many people employed outside their homes, for children at school, in day care or at college week-day, midday meals are usually eaten out.

Take-away foods and cheap eating-out establishments which are convenient are becoming increasingly popular with those who don't want to spend time shopping for or preparing and cooking food. The atmosphere and change of scenery can also be important for the aged and for people with little money or no paid work.

When eating food away from home everyone should, in an ideal world, be able to find meals or snacks which provide:

- plenty of bread, potatoes, rice or other starchy foods, especially those high in fibre
- plenty of fruit and vegetables
- low- and medium-fat foods, cooked only in a little fat
- low-sugar foods
- low-salt foods.

But is this possible?

We asked the participants in the survey whether their attempts at healthy eating were helped or hindered by available eating-out facilities.

While they were specifically trying to achieve the NACNE goals more than a third of the participants felt they had to cancel or avoid social eating out occasions as the food that would have been available would have made it impossible for them to achieve their targets. Also, of those who achieved or nearly achieved the goals over one-third decided they could not always eat their midday meal in their staff canteen and had to make other arrangements.

This is a sad but true indication of the poor facilities available for those who have decided they want to eat a more healthy diet.

The availability of eating-out facilities varies widely depending on many factors including whether the area is urban or rural; the type of local population and the size of the town but can be broadly divided into different categories, providing different types of food.

Cheap Restaurants, Cafés and Take-aways
Sizes and prices vary but these places are often used on a daily basis. The foods available also tend to vary on a regional basis.

Fish and Chip Shops
Almost all the food is deep-fried, often in batter – fish, sausages, fish cakes, chicken, spring rolls, chips, black pudding, haggis, tripe, spare ribs etc. Other foods usually include ready-made individual pies, pasties, patties, mushy peas and curry sauce. All but the last two are high in fat and often salt and have very little fibre. There are usually canned and bottled soft drinks (usually high in sugar) and pickles and sauces (high in salt) also available.

Some fish and chip shops are now diversifying to include kebabs, hummus and some Indian and Chinese dishes. On the whole it is fair to say that if you eat food from fish and chip shops more than once or twice a week on a regular basis it is very difficult to keep your fat intake down.

Kebab Houses
A selection of meats, grilled either on charcoal or by a gas burner is usually available. They are served in a pitta bread with a small portion of salad as a take-away. The meat is often fatty although some of the fat is lost during cooking. The bread is almost always low in fibre.

Cold dishes such as hummus (chickpeas and sesame seed paste – tahini), taramasalata (a fish roe paste) or tzatziki (a yoghurt and cucumber dish) are also often available. The tzatziki is low in fat and the hummus is a good source of fibre from the chickpeas it contains. Taramasalata is a high-fat choice.

Eat-in restaurants also usually serve rice and a greater variety of meat dishes.

Kebabs tend to be fatty but careful selection, e.g. of shish kebabs rather than doner kebabs may be a lower-fat choice. Maybe if demand were seen to be there kebab houses would start to use wholemeal pitta breads which are now available in supermarkets in some parts of the country.

Burger Bars

These vary widely in name but little in menu choice. A burger in a bun provides useful bread and meat and sometimes salad is included as a vegetable.

However, beef burgers, which mostly claim to be 100 per cent beef, can include more than 25 per cent beef fat, including suet. Some of this fat is lost in the cooking but not a significant amount. Burgers are also relatively high in salt. The buns (breadrolls) are usually of low-fibre white flour but one hamburger chain at least offers brown buns with their larger burgers. Some burgers include cheese, adding yet more fat to the existing fat and salt. Try to avoid these as a regular choice. Some burgers include a small amount of salad which will supply a little fibre and possibly some Vitamin C *if* the vegetables are not heated, cut up too small or left standing for too long. The chicken or fish burgers sometimes on offer are higher in fat than their unprocessed equivalents so regrettably these are not helpful in eating more healthily either.

There is not much help to be had from the other choices available. The composition of 'milk' shakes is unclear but the amount of milk present is questionable; they are certainly high in sugar and calories. Most burger bars sell deep-fried apple pies – also very high in fat.

Eating on a daily basis or even as frequently as two or three times a week from a burger bar would make it virtually impossible to make significant reductions in fat and salt intakes. Increasing one's fibre intake would also be tricky.

There is a real need for burger chains to look at their menus: to reduce the fat in their basic products; to offer wholemeal or brown buns as standard; to include more vegetable alternatives and to look at the possibility of including pulse dishes (for example, lentil or soya burgers) on their menus.

Baked Potato Shops

Baked potato shops are opening up all over the country after having started successfully in parts of Scotland many years ago.

Most shops sell large, baked potatoes with a wide variety of fillings which may be high or low in fat depending on the choice. The only problem can be that a large pat of butter or margarine is automatically put into the potato with the filling, usually without first asking the customer.

Perhaps the rule should be that the customer should opt *into* rather than *out of* having this extra fat. For the time being try and think ahead and say when ordering that you would rather have none added.

Sandwich Bars

Sandwich bars usually offer a wide and interesting range of fillings for sandwiches or rolls which are, in some parts of the country, brown or granary rather than white bread. Wholemeal bread seems rarely to be used. This may be because it breaks up more easily.

When bread and rolls are not spread with butter or margarine in advance why not ask for very little to be put on your bread. Fillings low in fat, salt and sugar are often available and fruit is frequently on sale.

Sandwich bars usually also sell cakes, biscuits, pastries and confectionery so a little restraint may be needed here.

Of all the relatively cheap eating-out places these can be the ones where the most healthy food is available for customers to choose. The main problem for people choosing is that, as with anywhere, it is not always easy to tell which of the foods are high or low in fat, salt, sugar and fibre.

Perhaps the labelling of menus would help people make more healthy choices.

Hot Dog Stalls

These are sometimes found in cinemas, or as mobile vans. They often double as ice-cream vans. The choice is very limited and is usually a frankfurter in a white bread roll with boiled onion rings and sauce. Like other sausages, frankfurters are high in fat and salt and the bread roll contains very little fibre.

Pizza Parlours
Pizzas are becoming increasingly popular in this country and, depending on the topping and type of flour used in the base, can provide plenty of fibre while being relatively low in fat and salt. Unfortunately, most pizza restaurants still use white flour in their dough although a few are beginning to introduce brown and wholemeal.

Indian Restaurants
These vary widely in the dishes they offer depending on which part of India, Pakistan or East Africa the restaurateurs originate from. There is always a wide choice of meat and vegetable dishes with rice and different types of breads. Although it can be possible to choose foods low in fat it depends to a large extent on the amount used in cooking as many meat and vegetable dishes are cooked in oil.

Although the rice served is usually polished, white and low in fibre, the vegetables, beans and lentils used are high in fibre.

Chinese Restaurants
Again, there is usually a wide variety of dishes that have varying amounts of fat and in addition are often high in sodium from added salt and monosodium glutamate.

The biggest challenge with all of these restaurants is avoiding fatty foods and finding foods high in fibre. It is not only hard to avoid the fat but it is virtually impossible to know either what fat is being used for frying or the saturated fat content of the food. Frequently vegetable oils are used for frying but these are not necessarily low in saturated fatty acids as they may contain palm or coconut oil.

Pubs and Other Restaurants
Many pubs now serve meals and it is becoming easier to get foods which will contribute to healthier diets. Nevertheless a whole range of high-fat, high-salt, low-fibre dishes still predominate. Some pubs are selling more salads and salad bars

are becoming increasingly popular generally. Unfortunately, salads are often automatically coated in dressings and mayonnaise which are all rich in fat.

Coffee Shops, Cafés and Tea Shops

These establishments in particular serve an invaluable social function. They are frequently used as a meeting place or somewhere to go for a little company.

Most of the produce tends to be high-fat, high-sugar and with an emphasis on serving tea, coffee, milky drinks, carbonated drinks and fruit squashes. Some such shops, of course, do sell sandwiches as well as breakfast or high-tea type meals such as fried eggs, bacon, baked beans or omelettes. Skimmed or semi-skimmed milk is rarely offered nor pure fruit juices or a range of sugar-free carbonated drinks.

A few establishments have ventured into selling wholemeal scones, wholemeal bread, sandwiches, salads, ploughmans and even fruit salad or muesli with yoghurt topping. This is a trend which needs to continue.

Some 'wholefood' type coffee shops or snack bars are offering a choice of fruit juices, herbal teas, decaffeinated coffee and sometimes low-fat milk. They may also sell sticky wholemeal cakes and biscuits. These can be full of fat and sugar so enjoy them occasionally but don't be fooled by their 'healthy' image!

The occasional 'naughty but nice' high-fat cream cake with a cup of coffee, whilst catching up on the news from a friend may do more good than harm. But for those who use these places regularly try to settle for just a drink free of sugar unless a quick meal is required. In this case look out for sandwiches and salads, poached eggs, baked beans and fruit items. It's worth enquiring about low-fat milk, wholemeal bread and polyunsaturated margarine.

Of the cakes: scones, choux pastry and bread-based items tend to be lower in fat than the pastries, making them a better choice.

Institutional Catering

Works' canteens, school canteens and eating facilities in other institutions such as hospitals, prisons, residential homes and so on, all vary and can be anything from domestic-sized kitchens serving a small number of people to large catering concerns with a number of kitchens and restaurants serving 3–4000 people a day.

The range of foods available obviously depends on the number of meals served and the facilities available as well as on the policy of the caterers. Happily some institutions, especially those in the public sector, are becoming more aware of the nutritional importance of what they are providing but unfortunately changes are slow.

It was interesting (and also a pity) to note in our survey that over one-third of the dietitians who managed to make significant changes in their diets felt they had to avoid eating in their hospital canteens in order to achieve those changes! They felt that with the foods available to them in the canteens they could not possibly reduce their fat or increase their fibre intake significantly.

More Expensive Restaurants

The type of food available in restaurants used purely for socialising or doing business is probably less important in health terms as fewer people eat in them often. However, for business people who have to entertain frequently it is often difficult to get food which is not smothered in butter, rich sauces or cream.

Eating out is probably one of the biggest obstacles to dietary change. Although many people eat out socially only rarely there is a large section of the population who rely routinely on food that they have no control over preparing.

The choice, although apparently considerable, is in fact very limited for someone who is trying to eat a more healthy diet. If we are serious about altering intakes of fat, fibre and salt in particular, there has to be a radical change in eating-out facilities, and healthy food has to be made available at a price people, especially those on low incomes, can afford.

Going Away

Going away may mean eating a lot of food prepared by others, with little choice over the amount of fat, sugar or salt you eat. For those who go away just for the occasional holidays or visits to friends and relatives the problem is quite different from someone who often travels away from home on business. The occasional traveller must first remember that healthy eating goals are achieved by everyday eating habits. Eating high-fat, high-sugar, high-salt or low-fibre foods more often when on holidays or staying with friends or relatives should have little effect on your long-term health. You may find that a holiday or break gives you a change in your everyday lifestyle and does you good. On the other hand, if going away means feeling constipated from the lack of fibre, tired and lethargic after high-fat foods and leaves with you a poor complexion and putting on weight – then you will need to take a different attitude. Your holiday will probably need a little more planning. Similarly, the regular traveller should also try to make some of these plans in order to maintain a healthy diet:

- Try to choose a hotel which offers wholegrain cereals, wholemeal bread, fresh fruit, low-fat yoghurts, potatoes other than chips and a good choice of vegetables.
- If you are highly motivated, plan to stay in a 'wholefood' guest house. These are advertised in health magazines. Although they all have different priorities with their cooking, some concentrate on wholegrain foods, others on 'natural' foods and they may or may not serve lower-fat foods; they are generally more discerning about their food.
- Try to have one meal a day of your own choice such as a picnic lunch or breakfast or sensibly chosen sandwiches from a take-away. Particularly when touring abroad where accommodation comes without breakfast, take your favourite cereal with you and buy some low-fat milk and fresh fruit. This makes a very easy picnic.
- Ask a guest house or hotel in advance for wholemeal bread or skimmed milk if you are staying for several days or warn your host of those eating habits that are important to

you. It may be helpful when staying with good friends or relatives to take one or two of the foods that are important to you such as a particular brand of spreading fat, wholemeal bread, low-fat milk (obviously judge the situation so you don't offend).

• It may be helpful to take unprocessed bran with you to add to fruit juice or soup. This can prevent constipation if wholemeal bread and wholegrain breakfast cereals are not available. Otherwise you may miss the fibre if you are used to a high level in your diet. Once the bowel is used to a high-fibre diet you will find that even a couple of days on white bread and other refined foods will make you constipated.

Adapting to the New Way of Eating

There are too many complex reasons why we all eat the way we do for anyone to recommend that we make the changes outlined in this section all at once. It is the gradual adoption of new habits that works best and it makes sense to start with those things that are easiest to change. You may wonder why the participants in our Study were asked to change over the period of one week. There is a simple answer to this – we wanted to know how to help you, the reader. Without any tried-and-tested teaching guidelines we know it would be difficult to help others to eat more healthily. Using dietitians and their households who have a good knowledge about food meant they could at least have a go at eating more healthily with little practical advice. It is likely that at least some of the participants who changed to healthier eating habits during the Study will return to some of their familiar habits but undoubtedly others will stick with certain of their changes for a life-time.

Here are some hints for adapting to the new way of eating painlessly.

• Think about changes you've made in your shopping and cooking over the past few years. If you are used to change then further change will be little problem to you.

- Go through all the foods in your larder. How many are on the suggested list of foods for your stock cupboard (see page 162 to 163)? Pick out those that are high in fat, sugar or salt or those that could be replaced by an unrefined variety.
- Decide which foods you have in stock will not be replaced and what you will buy instead.
- Then make a list of the meals you most regularly serve.
- Tick off the meals which fit in with the advice on fat, salt, sugar, fibre and alcohol.
- Put the remaining meals in order starting with the ones you or your family would find hardest to give up or eat less often.
- Each month or two try to introduce a new recipe that is low in fat and sugar and high in fibre and is tasty with little or no added salt. Let these recipes gradually replace the less healthy ones from the bottom of your list.
- Try to find ways of improving favourite recipes that are on your list – choose new cooking methods, for example baking instead of frying, or change ingredients – yoghurt instead of cream, a little oil instead of lard, wholemeal flour instead of white, or halve the sugar.
- Let the new shopping and cooking habits become familiar to you so that they are no more effort than before.
- Let one or two new habits settle before introducing a couple more.
- Get used to cooking and serving more potatoes, rice, pasta, vegetables, bread and cereals. You will need to use larger cooking pans and larger plates.
- We have mentioned several times that the new way of eating is bulkier. Be prepared to eat more starchy carbohydrates to compensate for the loss of some fat and sugar. Remember to drink more fluid with the higher-fibre foods.
- Slowly cut down the amount of fat, sugar and salt you add to foods and drinks. You then won't notice the change so much. For example, go in stages from two teaspoons of sugar added to a drink down to none after a few months. Similarly, gradually reduce the frequency of foods high in fat, sugar and salt.

Weaning

What is healthy for you is also healthy for babies. Sugary, fatty and salty foods are no good for them either.

- Start your baby around 4 months on your own puréed vegetables with no salt added – it should not be added to any of your baby's food.
- Next introduce breakfast cereal and sieved fruit with no sugar – this too should not be added to any of your baby's food. Allow him to enjoy the natural flavours of the foods rather than inflicting your taste for sweetness.
- Around 5–6 months introduce your home-cooked meat with vegetables, put through a mouli or liquidiser at first.
- Around 6 months give hard foods to chew on such as baked fingers of wholemeal bread or wholemeal toast, fingers of carrot or pieces of apple – always watch in case of choking.
- Soft-boiled egg yolk can be given.
- Introduce wholegrain cereals (without added sugar of course) and whole egg, scrambled or poached, and low-fat cheese. Banana is popular.
- Introduce fish (not smoked as this is too salty) and lentil soup or stew or your own cooked beans.

By 7 months your baby should be on a fairly mixed diet gradually taking food with more lumps. By 1 year the diet should resemble the rest of the family's.

- Always offer the savoury foods first. Also, use adult processed foods as little as possible, they are likely to be too high in fat, sugar and salt. Try to use the commercial baby foods only when you are travelling or when it is absolutely necessary.
- Avoid all commercial, sweetened drinks even if Vitamin C is added. Let your baby acquire the taste for water. This is the best drink to give in addition to milk. Alternatively give a little diluted, unsweetened fruit juice.
- Do not add unprocessed bran to your baby's food.
- There is no need to add margarine to bread but if you do, use a margarine high in polyunsaturated fat.

- Give your baby Children's Vitamin A, D, C Drops as advised by your health clinic.

Elderly People and the New Way of Eating

The dietary goals that the dietitians and members of their households put to the test were aimed at adults, and in particular the younger adult, although it is, of course, important for children to be brought up on a healthy diet. The new way of eating with the increase in fibre and reduction in fat and sugar is also richer in many nutrients.

In spite of this a slightly different attitude needs to be taken with the over-65s. The main reasons for altering the fat, sugar, fibre and salt content of the diet are to improve the quality of life and increase life expectancy. Altering these factors late in life will have far less effect than doing so in the teens or 20s. Guaranteeing adequate nutrients in the diet, however, becomes more of an issue as you get older. It is much more important to concentrate on choosing a wide variety of foods and eating regularly.

Only seriously cut down on fat and sugar if you are overweight or take rather a lot, otherwise just make a few modest changes. For example, if one of your meals is just bread, jam, cakes and biscuits, then you would be well advised to choose savoury foods and some fruit and salad instead. But taking only a little sugar in drinks, eating a few sweets or having a biscuit or cake each day are habits unlikely to harm you unless you carry excess weight or have diabetes. In fact, reducing your fat and sugar drastically, if you are not overweight, could cause unnecessary hunger and weight loss. You may find if you are elderly that you are unable to adjust by eating lots more bread, rice and pasta to make up for this lost energy. There is more sense, however, in making changes to increase your fibre intake. Regular, easy-to-pass motions make you feel much better. Make the changes gradually, or you may not reap benefits, just flatulence! Vegetables and fruits are rich in vitamins as well as fibre, so plan your meals using plenty of these. You may be advised to reduce your salt intake by your doctor because of high blood pressure, in this case the advice on salt in this book should be a help.

Lastly, there is alcohol to consider. Too much is not good for anyone at any age. Alcohol does not replace a meal – it is short of the nutrients you need for good health. More than a few drinks each week will bring you down both physically and mentally.

Weight Control and the New Way of Eating

One of the bonuses, if you are overweight, of a low-fat, low-sugar way of eating is that it will help you lose weight. This is because fat and sugar are both very concentrated sources of energy. Fat in fact is the highest source of calories, followed by alcohol so if you are overweight this is another reason you should go easy on the alcohol. The overweight, unlike those who are a healthy weight and are eating in this way, should not increase the amount of bread, potatoes, pasta and cereals they eat unless they were eating very little of these before. However, the overweight should choose high-fibre foods so as to minimise their feeling of hunger when reducing the fat and sugar they eat. Don't eat too much of the polyunsaturated oils and margarines. Try to cook without oil. If you use a fat on your bread it may be better to choose a low-fat spread, particularly if spreading thinly is difficult. You need to remember that fat is fattening whatever the type. To begin with you may not notice that you have decreased the amount you are eating. Most of the people in our Study found that they could not easily eat enough when cutting down on their sugar and fat intake so they showed just how easy it is to lose weight eating in this way! The menus below show the calorie intake of one participant eating normally and then eating to achieve the dietary goals.

Menu 1

Breakfast   2 slices of white bread spread with butter and marmalade
cup of coffee with a dash of whole milk and 2 teaspoons of sugar

Midday	A third of a 340g (12oz) quiche large helping of Brussels sprouts one small carton of cheesecake
Evening	250g (9oz) roast chicken leg frozen peas white sauce made from whole milk and margarine 1 wholemeal bap apple coffee with whole milk and 2 teaspoons of sugar
Snacks	2 small glasses of fresh orange juice 1 chocolate digestive biscuit 1 cup of tea with whole milk

Menu 2

Breakfast	2 Weetabix with skimmed milk 1 slice of wholemeal bread, spread with 1 teaspoon of low-fat spread 1 cup of coffee, with a dash of skimmed milk
Midday	2 slices of wholemeal bread with 2 teaspoons of low-fat spread 2 thin slices of boiled ham, lettuce, tomato and cucumber banana, with a small carton of low-fat natural yoghurt
Evening	Wholewheat lasagne with lentils as in Diary 2 medium-sized jacket potato cup of tea, with a dash of skimmed milk
Snacks	Apple cup of coffee with a dash of skimmed milk

The first menu provided 2000 calories and the second menu 1350 calories.

If you are trying to lose weight by eating in this new way, here are some tips that have been found to work. These are not like a slimming diet. For a start you will notice they are the healthy habits suggested for everyone throughout this chapter.

Milk and Cheese

- Where milk is used in a recipe, try skimmed milk instead. Beware, some dried milks have added vegetable fat.
- Cottage cheese or curd cheese are the lowest in calories. Dutch cheese and reduced-fat hard cheeses (e.g. Tendale, Shape, or own-brand reduced-fat cheeses) are lower in calories than other hard or cream cheeses.
- Grated cheese looks more and goes further than the same weight in a block.

Fats, Meat and Cooking Methods

- Fats are concentrated calories (as little as 15g provides 135 calories) so use less wherever possible in recipes and have fewer 'fry ups'.
- Use a low-fat spread, cottage cheese or other low-fat, skimmed milk soft cheese instead of butter or margarine, still spread thinly.
- Choose lean meat and pick cooking methods which remove most fat – grilling or baking. Food such as beef burgers and bacon can be grilled so that more fat drips away.
- Poultry is low in fat so try to choose it more often.
- Lightly brown mince first, and drain off the fat before continuing the recipe.
- Don't pre-fry meat and vegetables for stews – they can be cooked in a well-flavoured stock or with tomatoes. Alternatively brown the meat in a very lightly greased non-stick pan.
- Where possible skim the fat from stews and casseroles.
- Roast meat on a rack so that the fat drains away. Use vegetable stock, stock cubes or a gravy powder to make the gravy, rather than the pan drippings.
- Cooking with a non-stick pan or a wok will reduce the fat used in cooking. If necessary just grease it like a cake tin or use a spray-on fat.

- Remember that pâté and salami are high in fat and, therefore, high in calories.
- A pie with a potato topping is less fattening than pastry. There is no need to add butter to mashed potato or scrambled egg. Use skimmed or semi-skimmed milk instead, and cook scrambled egg in a non-stick pan.
- Snacks on toast, such as beans, scrambled egg, poached egg or cheese, do not need the toast buttered. They are less fattening choices than meat pies, pasties, sausage rolls or fried snack meals.

Fish

- Instead of fried fish try grilled or baked fish, adding vegetables, herbs and seasoning for flavour.
- Choose tinned fish in brine or tomato sauce rather than in oil. Otherwise drain off the oil.

Vegetables

- Eat more vegetables. Try vegetables that you do not normally eat. Try using onions, celery, tomatoes, carrots, green and red peppers, mushrooms, aubergines, marrow and courgettes. All of these are low in calories and add flavour to meals.
- Casserole of vegetables, which can include herbs, seasoning, onions, garlic or tomatoes can be a filling and tasty part of the meal.
- Use vegetable-based dishes more often e.g. stuffed marrow, peppers, tomatoes, potatoes. Flavoured cottage cheese makes a good filling for jacket potatoes.
- Use pulses and root vegetables to stretch a meat stew. They are cheaper than meat as well as being less fattening.
- Cook mushrooms and onions in lemon juice or stock rather than frying as they absorb a lot of fat.
- Choose clear or vegetable-based soups instead of thick, creamy soups. Try to add a few extra vegetables.
- Use more pulse vegetables. As lentils and beans are low in fat and contain lots of fibre use them to stretch a meat dish or to make a complete main dish.

Sauces and Dressings

- Use tomatoes and tomato paste in stews to make a thick, rich gravy.
- Thicken sauces and stews with cornflour rather than fat and flour.
- Yoghurt can be used instead of fresh or soured cream in savoury dishes. Add yoghurt when the dish has been taken off the heat, just prior to serving.
- Use plain yoghurt seasoned with salt, pepper, mustard, vinegar or lemon juice instead of salad cream, mayonnaise and salad dressings.
- Use plain yoghurt or buttermilk as a topping instead of cream or custard.

Sweet Foods

- Instead of buying sweetened fruit yoghurt add fresh fruit to natural yoghurt.
- Try fresh fruit or fruit canned in its own juice rather than tinned fruit in syrup. If you use artificial sweeteners, add after cooking.
- Some sugar substitutes contain sugar. These may be labelled as sucrose, dextrose, lactose, fructose, sorbitol – check the label before you buy.

Social Eating and Drinking

- A fatless sponge such as a Swiss roll is less fattening than a Madeira-type cake or Victoria sandwich.
- Whipped cream can be extended by adding whipped egg white.
- Eat a slightly smaller portion than you think you need! It might be helpful if you take a large helping of vegetables, leaving less room for other more fattening foods. It also draws less attention to your calorie counting.
- Always choose slim-line/low-calorie mixers if you are having a drink. Make sure any spirit drinks are a small measure.
- If you are a beer drinker, choose mild, light ale or ordinary lager and drink halves.
- If you like wine at a meal, ask for a second glass of water

(ordinary or carbonated mineral water). Drink your glass of wine at the end of the meal when it cannot be topped up!

● Raw carrots, celery, pepper and cucumber with yoghurt, cottage or curd cheese for dips or spreads make good 'nibbles' for a party. Flavoured cottage cheese can be a stuffing for celery pieces, or spread on to cucumber slices.

Flavouring

● Finally, try different flavours – sprinkle curry powder, garlic salt, crushed garlic, grated lemon or orange rind or mixed herbs over meat or fish before cooking. Add bay leaves, bouquet garni or thyme to stock for extra flavour.

Recipes

No book about food would be complete without some examples of what can be cooked at home. Clearly this is not a cookery book but eight recipes have been chosen with which many readers may be unfamiliar. They could be helpful when trying to follow a NACNE way of life.

Potato Salad

A delicious variant of an old favourite which can be modified for other salads.

Potatoes boiled in their skins
Dressing
3 parts yoghurt
1 part low-calorie salad cream
pinch curry powder (optional)

Mix dressing and use to coat sliced potatoes.

Apple and Raisin Tea Bread

Good for in-between-meals snacks.

225g (8oz) wholemeal flour
½ tsp ground mixed spice
1 tsp bicarbonate of soda
25g (1oz) soft vegetable margarine
1 medium-sized cooking apple

100g (4oz) stoned dates, chopped
100g (4oz) raisins
1 egg beaten
100ml (4fl oz) strong black tea
75ml (3fl oz) semi-skimmed or skimmed milk

Heat oven to 350°F/180°C/Gas 4.

Mix flour, spice and bicarbonate of soda in a bowl and rub in margarine. Peel, core and coarsely grate apple and stir into flour with dates and raisins. Make a well in the centre, add egg, tea and milk and mix until well blended. Pour into a greased 2lb loaf tin.

Bake for approximately 50 minutes until well risen and a skewer inserted in the centre comes out clean. Cool on a wire rack. Serve plain or spread with curd or cottage cheese.

Kidney and Bean Casserole   Serves 2

Shows how beans can be used to extend a meal.

175g (6oz) lamb's kidneys
15ml (1 tbsp) cooking oil
1 sliced onion (optional)
10g (⅓ oz) flour)

300ml (⅓pt) beef stock
5ml (1tsp) tomato purée
100g (4oz) baked beans
15ml (1 tbsp) natural yoghurt

Heat oven to 350°F/180°C, Gas 4.

Remove the skin from the kidneys, halve and remove the core.

Heat oil in a pan, add the kidneys and onions and cook for a few minutes. Stir in the flour, stock and tomato purée. Add the baked beans and mix well. Put all the ingredients into a greased ovenproof dish and place in oven for about 35 minutes or until tender. Stir in the yoghurt just before serving.

Lentil Roast   Serves 4

An appetising, low-fat alternative to meat. Any leftover can be used as a spread for sandwiches.

225g (8oz) lentils
275g (½pt) water
1 large onion, finely chopped
2 sticks celery or 1 large carrot, finely chopped
75g (2½oz) wholemeal breadcrumbs
3–4 tinned tomatoes, chopped

1 egg, beaten
15g (½oz) 1 tbsp oil
¼ lemon, zest and juice
mixed herbs and seasoning to taste
1 good tsp yeast extract
1 tsp curry powder (optional)

Wash lentils and cook in the water with the onion, celery or carrot in a covered pan for about half an hour.

When lentils are soft, stir in breadcrumbs, tomatoes, beaten egg, oil, zest of lemon, lemon juice, herbs, yeast extract and curry powder if used.

Put in a greased loaf tin and bake in oven for about 40 minutes at 350°F/180°C, Gas 4 until set and slightly browned.

Bean Cottage Pie   Serves 4

A tasty way of using beans.

675g (1½lbs) potatoes
5 tbsp milk
2 tbsp fresh parsley (if available)
2 tbsp oil
2 medium onions, thinly sliced
1 clove garlic, crushed
3 sticks celery, finely sliced
2 carrots, diced

Either 400g (15oz) tin kidney beans and 200g (7oz) tin butter beans (or use the 400g size)
or
225g (8oz) dried beans, soaked then cooked until soft
375g (14oz) tin tomatoes
1½ tbsp fresh herbs or 2-3 tsp dried herbs
3 tsp yeast extract
275ml (½pt) stock or water
pepper

Boil potatoes in their skins until tender. Then mash with milk and chopped parsley or some of the dried herbs.

Pre-heat oven to 400°F/200°C, Gas 6.

Heat oil in pan. Stir in onion, garlic, celery and carrot. Sweat in covered pan for ten minutes. Add the beans. Stir in tomatoes, remaining herbs, yeast extract, water and seasoning. Transfer to large ovenproof dish. Top with potato and decorate with a fork.

Bake in oven for 30 minutes until top slightly browned.

Wholemeal Scones   Makes 12

An enjoyable low-fat, low-sugar snack.

250g (8oz) wholemeal flour
2 × 5ml tsp baking powder
½ tsp salt
½ tsp cinnamon (optional)
50g (2oz) soft margarine
1 tbsp sugar

150g (5oz) natural yoghurt
40g (1½oz) dried fruit, e.g.
*   sultanas, chopped dates,*
*   currants, candied peel*
milk for brushing

Heat oven to 425°F/220°C, Gas 7.

Sift together flour, baking powder, salt and cinnamon in a large bowl. Rub in the margarine until mixture looks like fresh breadcrumbs and then stir in the sugar. Add yoghurt and fruit and lightly mix to a soft dough.

Roll out on a floured surface with a floured rolling pin to 2cm (1in) thickness. Cut with a fluted cutter. Place scones on a baking tray and brush with milk.

Bake for about 12 minutes until risen and golden brown.

Serve warm or sliced open with a little margarine or butter.

They can be stored in the freezer.

Oaty Fruit Crumble

Serves 4

Puddings can be healthy too!

500g (1lb) fruit – gooseberries, plums, pears, apples alone or with mixed spice, cinnamon, blackberries, blackcurrants or strawberries, apricots

50g (2oz) rolled oats
50g (2oz) wholemeal flour
40g (1½oz) soft margarine
25g (1oz) white or raw cane sugar

Heat oven to 375°F/190°C, Gas 5.

Wash and core fruit as necessary. No need to peel apples or plums. Lightly stew or bake in a little water. Place fruit in bottom of medium sized ovenproof dish.

Rub margarine into flour and oats with fingertips, until the mixture looks like fresh breadcrumbs. Mix in sugar and place crumble on top of fruit.

Bake in oven for about 35 minutes until browned and crispy on top.

Nut Loaf

Makes 4–6 slices

Try nuts for a main dish rather than just as a snack.

175g (6oz) nuts, e.g. hazelnuts, finely chopped
100g (4oz) fresh wholemeal breadcrumbs (or replace some with rolled oats)
1 onion, chopped
1 carrot or stick celery, chopped (optional)
15ml (1tbsp) oil

225g (9oz) tinned tomatoes with juice (if small tin used, make up to 9oz with water)
25g (1oz) wholemeal flour
1 egg, beaten
1 tsp mixed herbs
2 tsp Marmite or yeast extract

Pre-heat oven to 375°F/190°C, Gas 5.

Brown onion and carrot or celery in oil in a non-stick pan. Add chopped tomatoes (not juice), stir in flour and the tomato juice. Simmer whilst stirring for 2 minutes, add other ingredients and transfer to greased non-stick or lined loaf tin.

Bake for 45 minutes–1 hour until lightly browned and firm. Serve hot or cold.

Quick Meal with Pasta

A busy head teacher of a junior school in Luton offered his solution to eating healthily while living with the pressure of time. We reproduce it here because it has a lot to recommend it. Incidentally, he is proud to tell a gathering of a hundred or more pupils what he eats (very much in the NACNE style). His food clearly has multi-cultural appeal which is appropriate for his school of many races. The meal he suggests makes use of the one-pot idea and uses pasta which is quick to cook. It can be made as thick soup or a drier dish to eat off a plate.

Base	Variations	
sliced onion	*leeks*	*cheese*
garlic, finely chopped	*carrots*	*beans*
paprika	*spinach*	*cracked wheat*
pasta	*tomatoes*	

For **soup** consistency add plenty of water or vegetable stock and uncooked wholewheat pasta to the vegetable base of your choice, which has first been fried in a little oil. Cook until pasta is soft and then serve with grated cheese or yoghurt as appropriate.

For a **plate meal** cook the pasta separately then add to the base mixture which may need just a little water or vegetable stock added. Toss together and then serve with the yoghurt or cheese.

You can then try one of the following variations:

1 Sweat leeks and carrots with the base. (Serve this version with grated cheese.)
2 Sweat finely chopped carrots with the base and then add spinach (fresh or tinned) and tinned beans (not in sauce) or pre-cooked beans. A little low-fat yoghurt is stirred in just before serving.
3 Sweat carrots with the base and then add cracked wheat and some vegetable stock or tinned tomatoes. Cook until soft. Serve sprinkled with Parmesan cheese.

This is a quick meal for which you can think up your own variations – use your own favourite vegetables. Chopped nuts can be added just before serving or tinned fish used to replace the cracked wheat, or the beans. If you are not keen on following recipes rigidly, this suggestion should suit you.

CHAPTER SIX

Some Thoughts for the Future

Previous chapters have dealt in some detail with how individuals can choose to eat in a healthy way in keeping with the best scientific evidence and nutritional knowledge we have at the present time.

But all the responsibility should not be placed on individuals, or even on small groups of motivated people – at least not if change is to occur on any sort of lasting basis. Communities and society in general must choose to move towards healthier lifestyles and to create an atmosphere in which healthy, well-informed food choices become the norm.

So who does what to help or hinder the achievement of dietary goals? What recommendations can be made to make healthier eating an accepted part of modern lifestyles, without putting the total responsibility on the individual? No individual, government or food manufacturer can force people to eat healthily but they can make the task a lot easier! On the other hand we have to realise that most people don't buy food primarily with health in mind so there is a lot of work to be done to change public opinion in this sphere. Also, research shows that people's motivations to change to healthier ways of doing anything in life are very complex and very different.

What is needed then is a balance of changes from within the food industry itself, which will undoubtedly be forthcoming if there is a profit in it; from Government; and from the public as a whole. There are signs that such a balanced change is on the way.

The Government and its Influence on Food Production

There are many day-to-day aspects of life – and food is no exception – of which we tend to say, 'The Government should do something', and indeed the Government *does* have ultimate control over many services and activities that affect us all. When it comes to food we think it would be helpful if the Government took a greater responsibility to ensure:

- the consumer's right to know what goes into food – the ingredients and manufacturing processes – through adequate, informative labelling
- the right to know that food is safe from disease and contaminants through safety and monitoring, including the continuous monitoring and testing of food additives and pesticides
- the right to affordable, fair, prices.

Food Labelling
The NACNE and COMA Reports have accelerated interest in, and demand for, comprehensive and informative food labelling. There is an increasing awareness of the health implications of food and many people are getting into the habit of reading labels. What they find is not always useful. For those without a chemistry degree the strings of polysyllables in small print may mean very little or there may be no information on the label at all (which really lets one's imagination run wild!).

At present, we are advised to read the ingredients list, where ingredients appear in descending order of weight. This is informative to some extent, but is a rough estimate at best. For example, two ready-to-eat breakfast cereals may list sugar as the second ingredient. The cereal flake contains 7 per cent sugar, whereas the sugary 'kids' flake contains 30 per cent or more sugar. In other cases sugar or fat may be listed under several different names and therefore be at the bottom of the list of ingredients, e.g. sucrose . . . corn syrup . . . maltodextrins . . . honey. If added together to give the total sugar content this may well put sugar in the number one spot at the head of the list!

Clear statements backed by legislation are needed to inform us as to the exact amounts and proportions of some crucial components:

- total fat, as well as the amount and types of fat (that is, saturated and polyunsaturated)
- total carbohydrate as complex, unrefined starches and refined, simple sugars
- fibre
- salt
- sugar
- additives included during manufacture or packaging.

It is the Ministry of Agriculture, Fisheries and Food (MAFF) which researches, elicits discussion from key bodies and then finally proposes to Parliament regulations as to what labelling will appear on food packages and what claims can legally be made.

As a result of the impact of NACNE and COMA, scientists, consumer groups and MAFF, as well as a number of concerned groups, have called together working parties to look at the issue of labelling, starting with fat labelling in particular. The major issue to be resolved is deciding which information to include. A decision must also be made as to the single most comprehensive format in which to express this information.

This is a difficult area as there are so many possible solutions to the problem and the difficulties are not reduced by certain food companies protecting vested interests. The past ten years' experience of nutritional labelling in the USA has resulted in volumes of research on consumer understanding, or rather, lack of understanding. People do not want great lists of figures, 'E' numbers (codes for food additives) or percentages that seem to bear no relevance in terms of food intake or health. Similarly, people will become increasingly confused – and will ultimately reject – the variety of different formats that will proliferate if the whole thing is left to the discretion of individual manufacturers or retailers.

Giving adequate information on food additives that is helpful rather than alarming is another area of concern. A dilemma exists in that 'E' numbers do not mean very much to the majority of people. On the other hand, the name in full is not generally understood either. The booklet *Look at the Label* produced by MAFF is a good example of how such information can be presented in a form which is difficult to understand. This leaflet lists the names of the E numbers but gives no guidance as to the problems which have been associated with the use of some so we do not have all the available information to make an informed choice.

More of an issue, however, is the question of their use at all, alone or in combination with each other. Although this is not a subject that NACNE considered it is of such concern, especially in the matter of labelling, that we will look at it a little more under manufacturing because the decisions for the use of additives are usually made at this point.

Subsidies to Farmers

A substantial contribution to total fat intake in the British diet comes from animal sources: 27 per cent from carcass meats and meat products and around 30 per cent from dairy products.

The EEC subsidies that encourage farmers to produce animals to agreed specifications have changed for the better over the past five years. However, the subsidy system still leaves room for leaner animals to be encouraged. Very fat animals, such as traditional English breeds of pigs are no longer in demand and are not produced, having been replaced by hybrid pigs bred specifically for their leaner meat. The public's increasing demand for leaner cuts of meat has resulted in supermarkets (where an increasing number of retail meat sales are made) asking wholesalers to supply leaner carcasses. The suppliers in turn buy leaner animals from farmers. Many people feel this should be regulated further, so that the norm becomes lean-bred animals butchered to maximise leanness.

Beef and sheep carcasses are graded from fat classes 1 (the leanest) to 5. The subsidy is currently given to classes 2, 3 and 4. Class 4 is in need of revision as a result of nutritional recommendations and consumer pressures for lean meat. It has recently been suggested that this fat class subsidy be removed from lambs. There is a clear need for further research into the production of leaner animals through breeding, rearing and butchering techniques so as to ensure that meat consumed is as lean as possible while remaining palatable and acceptable to the public.

A relatively new cause for concern is the increasing fat content of chickens raised by battery farming operations. Traditionally promoted as a low-fat protein source, modern rearing and feeding methods used in poultry farming have resulted in a much higher fat content. As an increasing number of people are buying poultry from shops and supermarkets we would like to see a reversal of this trend for rapid fattening. Meanwhile, cooks will have to learn to cook poultry as they would duck – at lower temperatures for a longer period, allowing the fat to melt and drip away and be discarded.

The Butter Mountain

The butter mountain is ever-increasing – there were 928,000 tonnes of butter, valued at £2089 a tonne, in store in April 1985.* This mountain has come about as the result of, on the one hand, guaranteed prices increasing supply and on the other, falling consumer demand. Controls and quotas on milk production have started in an attempt to curb the problem but in the meantime promotional drives and subsidies attempt to rid the cold stores of this gross overproduction. The sheer size of the problem has convinced even the powerful milk lobby of the need for action.

The Government must seriously question the contribution this phenomenal amount of saturated fat and cholesterol is making to a diet already high in fat. We must continue to question the subsidised food given to those institutions such as schools and hospitals, where provision of such food goes against the health education efforts taking place within them. For example, we give subsidised milk to schools and subsidised butter to hospitals. As a result, hospitals may choose butter rather than other spreading fats because the former is cheaper to them.

*Intervention Board for Agricultural Produce (Butter Section) MAFF, 1985.

Food Manufacturers

We are often told that people are reluctant to change their eating habits and that any change can be expected to be very slow. Manufacturers have looked at this statement with disbelief. The ever-increasing array of foods on the shelves of the average supermarket has proved this is not the case. Exact figures are difficult to come by but in the early 1920s or 1930s there were around 900 food lines available; in 1970 this had increased to around 7500 and today most supermarkets carry over 10,000 lines. As these products would not be stocked unless they were bought we can see that people *are* prepared to change and to accept new products and eating patterns.

Snack meals and fast-food take-aways have grown rapidly over the past few years too, as have savoury snack foods such as crisps. It seems safe to assume that shoppers who buy these new lines have been influenced by the vast expenditure on advertising and marketing them.

The consumer ultimately foots the bill for this advertising and promotion. Advertising sets out to portray a particular product in the best light, either by emphasising its best features or by leading us to associate the product with pleasant or desirable feelings or activities. It is important to realise that many of the powerful messages that advertisements deliver are not about the product itself. They are about the promise of the sort of person you could be or would wish to be: the loving and loved mother; the accepted member of a fun-loving group of friends or the dazzling, attractive individual.

Not all products sold as 'healthy' in their advertising are in fact so. An example of this are the high-quality, motivating, 'health-provoking' advertisements produced for a major cereal company, whose products are high in sugar and salt, have added basic vitamins because the original ones have been refined out, and are high in additives to enable the product to be created in the first place.

There are thousands of good, healthy foods on the grocery shelves yet few are promoted with any nutritional expertise to adults and certainly not to children. The 'health' that is associated with a given product is part of the 'aura' surrounding the branded goods, not the outcome of the actual digestive process. A high-sugar muesli will supposedly make you bounce with health in the same way that a branded deodorant will make you a beautiful and rich businesswoman.

So we would like to see more honesty in advertising even though it would put an abrupt end to certain campaigns! The informative and truthful promotion of a product on health grounds is made much easier when the product is, in fact, a healthy one. This decision starts with the manufacturer.

The food that we eat has gone through a lengthy chain from its production by farmers to its sale through a retail outlet. The handling in between can involve anything from the basic process of placing the food into some form of container for distribution, through the many ways that it can be processed, refined, altered and so on into its final, saleable form. It is estimated that around 75 per cent of the food we eat has been processed in some way. This can range from simple procedures such as the grinding of wheat into flour through to the new techniques that turn food into food 'products'. To use the example of wheat, this basic nutritious food can be crushed, inflated, refined, enriched, coloured, stabilised, emulsified or in many other ways transformed into a variety of 'novel' products.

This constant innovation helps to keep the food industry growing and profitable. Companies must maintain or improve their market share to continue to finance their present level of business; to re-invest in potential expansion; and to make a profit.

The financial risk involved in researching, producing and marketing an unsuccessful food product is a real one. Many large food manufacturers develop new products on a regular basis, a few of which make it to the supermarket shelves, with even fewer remaining as established lines.

Currently the tide of fashion is running in favour of health and healthy foods. As this is also conducive to profit as a result of growing consumer demand, manufacturers can be expected to respond with the development of new products – most with higher profit margins.

The number of people concerned about nutritious food is

growing and they are demanding real choice at affordable prices. We would like to see a critical review of the existing food supply and how food might be re-formulated to better fit into NACNE-type goals.

The lack of suitable convenience foods was a major problem for many of our participants. Many people condemn all convenience foods or pre-prepared foods as inferior. In fact, there *should be* nothing inherently wrong with convenience foods – it is the proportion of fat, sugar, fibre and salt that matters and not necessarily the form that you choose to eat it in. Generally, and unfortunately, at the moment it is likely that if you rely on the currently available range of convenience foods, you will be less likely to eat a healthy diet along the lines recommended by NACNE.

Frozen foods are an enormous area for future development in convenience foods. Although many frozen products can suffer when it comes to flavour and texture, nutritionally they are often as good as fresh. Fruits and vegetables may even retain *more* nutrients because they are packaged very soon after harvesting. Although frozen fish accounts for the majority of purchased fish (excluding that sold in fish and chip shops) even this is a small amount. The current cost of frozen meals is high and most are made up in rich sauces and are high in fat and additives. Frozen foods in boxes are usually generously packaged but with meagre contents – a large illustrated packet leads you to overestimate the value of a very shallow box.

Technological breakthroughs that can generate a whole array of convenience foods and the ability to adulterate basic food products have far outstripped legislation. To use meat as an example: many new meat products call for the addition of up to 20 per cent water and moisture-retaining polyphosphates to hold this water in. Trading standards officers are increasingly concerned about the progressive adulteration of meat by the use of 'improvers' and 'extenders' for extra profit. Milk protein can allow an extra 13 per cent brine solution to be added to hams and at the same time mask the salty taste. Meat is already broadly defined to include choice cuts such as ear, lip, nose and rind! Adequate and comprehensive labelling is the only solution to complete consumer awareness but a progressive review of legislation is really what is needed so that enforcement agencies can operate as quickly as technological developments occur.

Just as legislation is not tight enough to control current and future developments, other food legislation and 'manufacturing codes of practice' can restrict development in a healthier direction. Margarine, for example, has to be 80 per cent fat to fall within the legal definition of margarine. When 40 per cent fat margarines first came out they were illegal; because they are now renamed 'low-fat spreads' they are allowed. Jam must contain 60 per cent sugar by law and only under the guise of 'low-sugar preserves' can lower-sugar products be developed. This type of legislation or manufacturing agreement, long ago introduced to protect the consumer against the adulteration of foods can inhibit potential new product development or the re-formulation of existing products along healthier lines.

There is a real need for the encouragement and development of a choice of healthy alternatives to many existing basic commodities at a mass-market price and with widespread availability. Manufacturers are responding. There are many products that already meet the following recommendations but most tend to be marketed to the health-conscious middle class who are prepared to pay more for health. Unfortunately, in many cases claims are spurious, such as a biscuit with a 'health image' containing some wholegrain flour but still containing a high proportion of saturated fat, sugar and salt.

Food	Development required
Breakfast cereals	High-fibre, low-salt, low-sugar and low-fat, fewer additives and less refining
Bread, baked goods	High-fibre, low-salt, low-sugar and low-fat
Meat	Leaner cuts and products low in fat and salt

Fish	Tasty low-fat, low-salt fish dishes to encourage an increase in the present low fish consumption
Dairy products	Low-fat and low-salt
Cheese	A larger and tastier variety of low-fat, low-salt
Tinned fruit	Without added sugar
Tinned vegetables	Without salt
Condiments and sauces	Reduced sugar and salt
Convenience foods (savoury, sweet and snacks)	A variety of tasty, frozen, chilled or tinned ready-to-eat healthy alternatives as outlined in previous chapters

Food Retailers

For many shoppers, the most visible link in the food chain is the retailer – either the small shop, the supermarket, the specialist outlet or the health food shop. You don't have to go to a 'health' shop to get healthy food, although many carry a greater variety of grains, pulses and various lower-cost herbs and spices than do general outlets. Remember that 'healthy' foods may not in fact turn out to be so healthy when you read the labels. All that is brown is not necessarily beautiful and many processed products are high in honey or brown sugar, which are equally bad for your teeth. The health food market is growing rapidly and it is possible to pay more for a product packaged in a 'health-inspiring' pack than if you buy the same item in a supermarket chain. This can be confusing to the busy shopper – and that is most of us!

As with manufacturers, retailers, large or small, are profit-driven. Retailers stand to make money from consumer trends, just as they will fail to profit or retain their market share if they fail to supply or stock items that are in demand.

We suggest that readers demand that healthier items be carried by their local shop. Will they, for example, stock more wholemeal bread or skimmed milk so that supplies don't run out before working people get to the shops after 4.30 or 5.00 pm? Would they stock cottage cheese without E412, E415 and E410! This calls for a certain level of assertiveness on the part of the individual, besides running the risk of being welcomed one day and treated as the local pest the next!

Generally, shops will carry items they know will sell to their regular clientele. Ideally shop owners and managers could instigate schemes whereby healthier food is readily available, promoted and prominently displayed in preference to less healthy alternatives. Questions arise as to the problems this could cause for large suppliers of less healthy products!

We would like to see retailers taking a stronger role in nutrition education programmes within shops in a variety of ways. The following suggestions and examples may be useful ideas in shops and supermarket chains:

- Provide information sheets promoting healthy choices at the cash-till or on the shelves.
- Provide clear, informative, simple food labelling. Increasing numbers of retail chains in the UK are labelling their own brands. Ideally this will eventually spread to all foods!
- Use healthy foods as loss leaders to keep their prices comparable with less healthy alternatives.
- Use marketing techniques to promote the sale of more healthy foods.
- Follow the example of some stores in the USA by promoting consumer involvement to disclose useful findings, such as the sugar content of breakfast cereals.
- Employ dietitians and/or home economists to answer consumer questions and to plan promotions and in-store tasting sessions on healthy foods and new ways of cooking.

Supermarket layout is carefully designed to influence what people buy. Shoppers are often led through impulse items such as sweets and biscuits to get to the basic commodities such as dairy products, fruit and vegetables and meat. Sweets are still placed at check-outs, waiting for hungry shoppers, although some retailers have announced that they will discontinue this. Children's cereals and biscuits are often placed at child's-eye level, so that shoppers with children are vulnerable to the impulse buying of sweets, snacks and other TV-advertised foods.

The Catering Industry

Many participants found their attempts to follow the NACNE guidelines were made very difficult when dining out in restaurants and when relying on canteens, cafés and take-aways. There is a spiralling growth of fast foods and quick take-away meals. Fast food restaurants have shot up from a few in the 1940s and 1950s to thousands today. Those who oppose this trend say that foods eaten on the run are likely to be 'junk' foods, high in calories, sugar, salt and fat and low in fibre and other nutrients.

Once again, restaurants are commercial ventures and can only survive where they have a steady supply of satisfied customers. Canteens in workplaces are a separate issue as often their 'customers' have no alternative unless they bring their own food.

Many suggestions included in previous chapters can be incorporated when eating out. If you are dining out socially or entertaining someone there is often a choice of outlets allowing you to select the restaurant most conducive to your needs. When the number of restaurants is limited, or if eating out is a routine, necessary part of your lifestyle, this is not so easily done. The onus lies with the catering industry to take a responsible role and to set standards for itself in the area of nutrition. Training colleges and schools which educate catering staff, chefs, cooks' assistants, and all basic preparation courses in schools and food administration courses should place more of an emphasis on nutrition principles – both their theory and practical application. Change is more likely to take place where those responsible for running food outlets and for preparing food are themselves well informed and personally interested.

A sensible first step is to take a new look at menus and food preparation techniques as well as the standard ingredients used in catering outlets. Once this has been carried out the following changes could be put into action:

- The substitution of healthier ingredients in recipes. Wholemeal flour substituted for white; an oil high in polyunsaturates instead of saturated cooking fat; low-fat milk rather than full-fat; and so on. In this way the menus and dishes are kept outwardly similar. If such changes are brought in slowly then alterations in taste will be kept to a minimum and remain acceptable to customers. The results of our survey would suggest that such changes could well bring in new customers.
- Reviewing handling and cooking techniques can bring about improvements – less frying and more grilling; leaving fats such as butter or salad dressing as something the consumer chooses to add rather than adding it 'at source'.
- The addition of new dishes, be they main dishes, side dishes or desserts, where healthy alternatives are lacking. Most pasta and rice-based dishes, and fish meals that are not fried would improve many meat-based menus, as would vegetable selections and the availability of wholemeal breads on menus where these are not previously available.
- Standard portion sizes could also be reviewed. Many a 'ploughman's lunch', for example, has a large hunk of cheese but very little bread.
- Once a menu has been assessed, with appropriate changes made, these healthier alternatives can be indicated in a simple, uniform format. Thus existing dishes become healthy and well informed customers can make their own choices.

The Crest chain of hotels in the UK have their Lifespan menus available for residents to choose from in which healthy choices are indicated. Restaurants in the Minnesota Heart Health Programme in the USA have a system in which small heart signs are used to indicate 'heart-healthy' choices.

The catering industry, and especially the Government-influenced sectors (which feed more people than any other single caterer), can, by demanding healthier mass-market food, put pressure on the food industry to supply it. Once a given food is then being manufactured for so large a customer it will not be long before it can be found in supermarkets everywhere. Also, the vast numbers of people who are fed by Governmental catering services will be only too willing to go out and buy it if they have enjoyed it. Such an approach also has the advantage of making the healthier food available quickly at a mass-market price rather than at a 'health food' price.

The above recommendations are equally relevant to canteens servicing industry and businesses. In these cases it is more crucial that a real choice be offered, as people may have no other option. Many district health authorities are implementing Healthy Eating Policies and liaising with social services, education services and local industry to promote a wider nutritional awareness. Where such ideas are adopted this will involve extensive education for staff and consumers. Once again choice and variety of foods needs to be encouraged.

Food companies are beginning to see that NACNE is here to stay and will increasingly mean more profits. Food manufacturers and retailers are realising that the public are increasingly involving health in their reasons for choosing foods. They are also aware that the public needs to know more about what food contains.

What is needed is for more dietitians to be employed from the inside, that is within food companies where all the decisions are being made about our food and health, rather than just acting from the outside, in educating the public. Dietitians working from within food manufacturers and retailers can then be involved in decisions on food quality when such questions are raised as whether to add more salt or fat to a product to improve its shelf life, or to advise on new product development. All the factors can then be weighed up including the nutritional ones, and satisfactory compromises can be found. The nutritionist could also be of value to the company in pointing out the merits, for example, of a polyunsaturated fat added to a product instead of a saturated kind. These merits would be invaluable in advertising and public relations drives

– helping NACNE to mean profit to both the health of the nation and the food industry.

The suggestions we have made in this chapter are not meant to be definitive but we hope they are fairly comprehensive. Clearly, there are hundreds of different things that could be done by the Government and the food industry to help make healthy eating a lot easier than it is. Indeed, even since we first started work on the Study more changes have been suggested and improvement is occurring all the time.

Appendix:
Some of the Materials Used in the Study

PERSONAL DATA – *COMPLETE AT THE BEGINNING OF THE WEEK*

The following personal data is required to complete an evaluation of your nutritional status. All information will be strictly confidential. Please answer all questions.

1 Age ..... years
2 Height ..... ft ..... ins   OR ..... cms
3 Weight ..... st ..... lbs   OR ..... kgs (Beginning of
                                                  the week)

4 Would you describe yourself as:
      1 Relatively active
      2 Moderately active   ( )
      3 Very active
5 Would you call your frame size:
      1 Large
      2 Medium   ( )
      3 Small
6 Are you: Omnivorous   ( )
                                    Vegetarian   ( )
                                    Vegan   ( )
                                    Other   ( )
  If other, please describe _____

_____

7 Do you follow a therapeutic diet? Please specify: Yes/No   ( )

_____

8 Do you regularly eat three meals a day?   Yes/No   ( )
9 Are there any foods that you do not eat for religious or moral reasons? If yes, please comment: _____

_____

10 Do you usually add salt to your food at the table or in cooking?
                                                Yes/No   ( )
11 Do you smoke?   Yes/No   ( )
    If yes, how many cigarettes/cigars/oz tobacco per day?
                                                (   )
12 Do you have any family history of heart disease?
                                                Yes/No   ( )
13 Do you suffer from raised blood pressure? i.e., above 160/95mm Hg   Yes/No   ( )
14 Do you regularly (at least twice/week) take any form of physical exercise (e.g., jogging, squash, cycling)   Yes/No   ( )
15 Do you consider yourself to be under more than usual emotional or work-related stress?   Yes/No   ( )
16 Do you put on weight easily?   Yes/No   ( )
17 Are you aware of any health problem which might be related to, or the treatment of which may effect your nutritional require-ments?   Yes/No   ( )
    If yes, please give details _____

_____

18 Do you regularly take any vitamin/mineral preparation?
                                                Yes/No   ( )
    If yes, please state names and, if possible, contents _____

_____

19 Are you pregnant? If yes, how many weeks? ..... wks
                                                Yes/No   ( )
    Are you breast feeding?
                                                Yes/No   ( )

QUESTIONNAIRE I – COMPLETE AT END OF WEEK

The following data is needed to investigate the inter-relationship between eating habits and lifestyle. Please tick the relevant bracket, or comment as appropriate.

1 Do other members of your household eat similar meals to yourself?

Yes ( )
No ( )
N/A ( )

2 Do you think that the availability of suitable recipes affects your efforts to eat a healthy diet?

Yes ( )
No ( )
Uncertain ( )

Please comment _____

_____

___

3 Where was the shopping done for the food you *ate* during the weighed food survey?

Please indicate the shop used most frequently as 1, the next as 2, etc., for all shops used.

	SCORE
Supermarket	( )
Small general grocers	( )
Traditional shops e.g. butcher, baker, greengrocer	( )
Market	( )
Health Food Shops	( )
Wholefood grocers	( )
Ethnic shops i.e., Indian, Chinese	( )
Other (please specify) _____	

4 Do you think that the availability of suitable pre-prepared foods affects your efforts to eat a healthy diet?

Adversely ( )
Advantageously ( )
Uncertain ( )
Not at all ( )

5 How long each day do you spend in preparing the food you ate, and clearing up? Exclude time spent recording weights. Please give your best estimate.

(Mins)

6 Are there any factors that limit the enjoyment of your diet? e.g., time, availability of foods, cost, knowledge about food, etc.

Yes ( )
No ( )
Uncertain ( )

Please comment _____

_____

7 Do you think the weighing and recording of your food intake altered your normal eating habits during this survey?

Yes	( )
No	( )

Please comment _____

_____

8 Do you agree with setting dietary goals for a population?

Yes	( )
No	( )

Please comment _____

_____

9 Weight at the end of the week
..... st ..... lbs   OR ..... kgs

COMPLETING YOUR 7 DAY FOOD DIARY

The purpose of this food diary is to estimate your dietary intake, both in quantity and quality. The degree of accuracy relies on the completeness of your record. This cannot be over-emphasised.

Choose a week, within the next three weeks, that you anticipate will be representative of your usual eating pattern. A seven day record is generally assumed to give more valid results.

Write down EVERYTHING that you eat and drink during the seven days. Try to do this after each meal or snack while the information is still fresh in your mind. Please specify the following:

H – Food or drink prepared at home, or packed and taken to work
C – Purchased at office/hospital/work canteen
F – food prepared by friends/relatives
R – restaurant, café or take-away including shop-bought snacks for immediate use, e.g., confectionery, sandwich, fruit, drink

Quantities of food must be weighed in grams (or ounces), to the nearest 5g (or ¼oz). Estimated weights should only be given when absolutely necessary. Please indicate estimated weights with an 'E', e.g., 50g E. Where weights are stated on bars of chocolate, crisp bags, cans of juice, please use them.

Please record *cooked* weights of foods.

Please record *brand* of oil and fats. This affects the calculations significantly.

Please give a DETAILED description including name and/or brand name of foods eaten – for example:-

Bread –   is it white, brown, wholemeal, granary etc?

Meat –   is it leg, shoulder, chop etc? Is it lean and fat? Is it roast, grilled, boiled, fried, casseroled? If fried, in what type and brand of oil/fat? If casseroled, what other ingredients were used?

Potato –   boiled, mashed, chipped, roast, sautéed? If mashed, was milk and butter or margarine added? What brand was the oil/fat.

Certain foods, e.g., butter, margarine, sugar, can be weighed at the *beginning* of the week and *end* of the week. Set aside a weighed amount of the food for your own consumption only. Milk can be measured on a daily basis if preferred.

Your accuracy helps minimise error in coding

Enjoy your week!

SAMPLE OF A FIRST NUTRITION ASSESSMENT
(FOR A MALE PARTICIPANT)

Dear Participant,

Thank you for recording your food intake and for answering the questionnaire. We have now evaluated this information and the following recommendations are based on what you have told us. The guidelines used for this assessment are those of the expert committees from the DHSS (1977) on nutrient intakes, FAO/WHO (1977) on dietary fats, WHO (1982) on the prevention of heart disease and the National Advisory Committee on Nutrition Education (1983).

Section 1. YOUR PERSONAL DATA. The data you reported is shown below:

Age	31 years
Height	173 cms
Weight	60.0 Kg
Frame size	Medium

According to the Metropolitan Life Insurance Company (1983), your weight is 8.5 per cent below the lower limit desirable (65.6 –71.0kg) for your height and frame size.

Section 2. YOUR DIETARY/NUTRIENT BREAKDOWN.
The nutrients provided by the food and beverage items you reported
are shown below. The recommended daily intake for a group of
persons your age, sex and activity level is compared below with your
average daily intake for the period you recorded:

Nutrient	Unit	Recommended Daily Intake (RDI)		Your Average Daily Intake	Action Required
Energy	Calorie	2510.0		2306.7	
Protein	g	63.0		78.5	
Fat (Total)	g	<30% Kcal		95.0	
Carbohydrate (Total)	g	###		297.0	
Sugars	g	###		166.8	
Fibre	g	30.0	NACNE	22.6	Increase
Potassium	mg	###		3255.2	
Calcium	mg	500.0		955.4	
Iron	mg	10.0		13.0	
Zinc	mg*	15.0		10.7	
Sodium	mg	<3600	NACNE	2929.4	
Vitamin A (RE)	mcg	750.0		981.9	
Carotene	mcg	###		2366.0	
Vitamin D	mcg	Sunlight!		5.4	
Vitamin E	mg*	15.0		6.0	
Vitamin B12	mcg*	3.0		3.9	
Riboflavin	mg	1.6		2.2	
Niacin (NE)	mg	18.0		38.2	
Vitamin C	mg	30.0		91.7	
Vitamin B6	mg*	2.0		1.4	
Folic acid	mcg	300.0		158.8	
Cholesterol	mg	<300		373.6	
Saturated fat	% of Kcals.	<10	NACNE	15.9	Decrease
Essential PUFAs	% of Kcals.	>3.0		5.4	
P/S Ratio		1.0		.3	
% Kcalories from protein				13.6	
% Kcalories from fat		<30	NACNE	37.1	Decrease
% Kcalories from carbohydrate				48.3	
% Kcalories from added sugars		<10	NACNE	15.0	Decrease
% Kcalories from alcohol		<8.0		1.0	

[### no recommended figure has been set, * Nat. Res. Council (USA) rec.]

Section 3. ASSESSMENT OF YOUR DIETARY INTAKE

Although the assessment provides you with information about most of the nutrients thought to be important to health, the purpose of this exercise is to consider the NACNE long term guidelines only. Nutrient requirements can vary considerably from individual to individual. We have chosen + or − 10% as the arbitrary upper and lower limits to the NACNE recommendations, within which no action need be taken. Dietary evaluations cannot be taken as an absolute indication of adequate nutrition. They do, however, provide evidence of probable dietary inadequacies or excesses and help in assessing the need for appropriate intervention programmes. Your calorie intake was below the DHSS recommendation and your weight was also below the desirable range for a person of your frame size and height. There are, of course, wide variations in energy requirements between individuals and only you will know if you are wasting away or maintaining good health! NACNE does not make specific recommendations on calorie intakes but at low calorie intakes there is a tendency for the intakes of certain other essential nutrients to suffer. Your intakes of zinc, vitamins E, B6 and folic acid were low (and your cholesterol intake a little high) in comparison with International recommendations and we thought we should draw this to your attention. We did not include the Plurivite in the analysis so that you could judge for yourself whether they were necessary or not.

As part of a health care programme we would suggest the following adjustments to your diet to bring it in line with the guidelines of the National Committee on Nutrition Education:-

SODIUM: While your sodium intake was below the long term NACNE recommended upper level of 3600 mg/day, the analysis does not take into account salt added in cooking and/or at table. As you state you do add salt it is quite possible that your total intake is in excess of 3600 mg.

Animal experiments have shown that modest intakes of sodium, though higher than naturally occurring in the animal's food, can lead to hypertension in those who are genetically susceptible. It has also been demonstrated that a fall in blood pressure occurs when humans are given a diet low in sodium and that high salt intakes are associated with hypertension and stroke. Current recommendations suggest that salt intake should be reduced to less than 5g per day, a fairly radical reduction from the present estimated average British intake of 12g/day. Such a drastic reduction will obviously necessitate major changes in food manufacture but in the meantime you are advised to reduce the amount of salt used in cooking and at table to a minimum with an ultimate aim of eliminating added salt completely from your diet. Try herbs and spices or lemon juice to substitute for the added flavour given by salt. Alternatively, taste food in its natural state again!

FIBRE: Your fibre intake is below the recommended intake of 30gms per day. Since fibre is intimately associated with foods providing many vitamins (folic acid, thiamin, niacin, vitamin C, carotene, vitamin B6) a low fibre diet is often a predictor of a low vitamin intake. Constipation is a common problem and the addition of extra fibre in your diet often helps to prevent it. It is also thought to prevent certain intestinal diseases such as diverticulitis and cancer of the colon. There is evidence that plasma cholesterol levels fall with diets high in fibre. The best sources of fibre include wholemeal bread, bran and oat cereals, vegetables and fruit.

SUCROSE: This analysis includes all refined sugars e.g. sucrose, and glucose. NACNE suggests that sugar in the form of table sugar, confectionery, snacks and soft drinks should be restricted as much as possible, particularly between meals in an attempt to avoid a) obesity and b) dental caries. Present evidence suggests that sugar contained within meals seems to be less cariogenic than that consumed between meals.

ALCOHOL: The NACNE recommendations on alcohol intakes refer to 20g per day consumption in the 1960's; but this is a mean value for all which includes infants, children and those who do not drink. We suggest a realistic interpretation of this might be that it would be wise to keep alcohol consumption to below 8% of your energy. Your intake therefore, is within a satisfactory limit.

FAT: Your intake is above the NACNE recommendation that fat should contribute less than 30% (long term guideline) of your calorie intake. In the interest of preventing coronary heart disease your total fat should be reduced, particularly by reduction of the saturated fats.

SATURATED FAT: There is a strong correlation between saturated fat intakes, blood cholesterol levels and the incidence of heart disease. Saturated fats increase platelet stickiness and at high intakes, are atherogenic. There is a universal recommendation that saturated fats should be decreased to about 10% of the dietary energy. Your intake was higher than this and we would recommend that you reduce, still further if you have already done so, your use of foods rich in saturated fatty acids. These include the visible fat on meat, full fat cheeses, butter, hard margarines, blended vegetable oils, shortenings, lard, suet and foods made with these, such as biscuits, pies, sausages, pastries and cakes. It is unusual for cream to be eaten regularly and is seldom a problem but 60% of the fat on the top of the milk is saturated and it is advisable to use semi-skimmed or skimmed milk which is now generally delivered by the milkman.

Your P/S ratio was too low at 0.35; NACNE considers that health benefits would arise from a ratio in the region of 0.6–1.0. The P/S ratio refers to the balance of essential fatty acids (EFA) to the non-essential, saturated fats. This has been found to be a useful concept in so far as saturated fats compete with the utilisation of the essential fatty acids. A high intake of saturated fat increases the requirement for EFAs. The EFAs are needed for structural lipids (cell membranes) and for cell regulation via their prostaglandins and leukotrienes. They are especially relevant to the vascular, reproductive and immune systems. Parent essential fatty acids are linoleic and alpha-linolenic acids. Linoleic acid is found in seeds and seed oils and alpha-linolenic acid in dark green leafy vegetables where it is associated with vitamins E, C and folate. Foods rich in the EFAs are whole seed foods, beans, nuts, dark green vegetables, fish and marine foods. Meat should be a rich source but is often so fatty that it provides a high proportion of saturated fats instead; however, game meat and very lean meat is a good source of EFA rather like fish. Try the French practice of regularly using oil and vinegar with green salads which has the merit of increasing your intake of both families of essential fatty acids. Dietary moves in this direction will also increase the intake of trace elements and a number of vitamins (e.g. E, folic acid, Zn).

Section 4. PREVENTION OF HEART DISEASE
Since heart disease is the most common cause of premature death in Britain with one in four men having a heart attack or stroke by retirement age, it is appropriate that special attention should be paid to the known risk factors. Population based action on diet, blood pressure, smoking and exercise in Finland, the USA, Canada and Australia has been associated with a significant reduction in the incidence of CHD in these countries. All the International and National Committees, including NACNE and the DHSS (1984) have agreed to the need to reduce total fat intake and particularly the intake of saturated fats. Assuming a reduction in the general amount of fat and particularly in saturated fats, NACNE considered that an increase in the ratio of essential to saturated fatty acids from the present low levels to the region of 0.6 to 1.0 could be beneficial.

The following table considers the lifestyle choices that you have made and your family history that should be taken into account when planning your personal health care programme.

1. DIET		See the dietary recommendations above, paying special attention to those on fat and salt.
2. SMOKING	NO:	A health bonus! Your risk of dying from a heart attack is ten times less than that of a heavy smoker.
3. FAMILY HISTORY OF CHD	YES:	No-one can choose their genetic make-up but it can be taken as an early warning light and preventative steps are particularly important in your case.
4. OVERWEIGHT	NO:	A health bonus!
5. EXERCISE	NO:	In a study carried out in America, the risk of death from ischaemic heart disease was found to be almost three times greater in inactive men than in those who participated in some form of regular exercise. Exercise also improves general physical well-being. It is important to take part in some form of regular exercise which you enjoy and which increases your pulse rate.
6. STRESS	NO:	A health bonus! While stress may not cause the disease to the arteries and blood which leads to heart attacks, it is believed to be important in the timing of an attack.
7. HYPERTENSION	NO:	A health bonus! Keep it that way.

Section 5. SUMMARY OF RECOMMENDATIONS
The following recommendations are aimed at providing you with the best information maximising your chances of good health and preventing illness.

YOUR DIET: should be adjusted as follows:

Increase . . .

* Fibre – e.g. wholemeal bread and flour, 'high' fibre breakfast cereals, fruit and vegetables.

We suggest you may be able to cut down a little on . . .

* Added sugar, also high sugar desserts, drinks and confectionery.
* Salt – Try to avoid adding extra salt to your food, even in cooking!
* Fats Particularly saturated fats . . . e.g. fatty meat, full fat cheeses, whole milk, butter and cream. You should replace some of the saturated fats with polyunsaturated fats.

YOUR LIFESTYLE: We recommend you consider the following lifestyle changes:

* Take more regular exercise.
* Enjoy life! Remember you will enjoy it more in full health and only YOU can help ensure this!

We hope you have enjoyed participating in this assessment of your nutritional status and we wish you the best of health in the future.

This analysis is provided by the Flora Project for Heart Disease Prevention, using data supplied by the Department of Biochemistry and Nutrition at The Nuffield Laboratories of Comparative Medicine, McCance & Widdowson's 'The Composition of Foods' and the American Department of Agriculture.

The Flora Project for Heart Disease Prevention
25 North Row
London W1
Tel 01-499 0414

The Flora Project for Heart Disease Prevention is a service provided by Van den Burghs & Jurgens Ltd.

QUESTIONNAIRE II
PLEASE COMPLETE THIS AT THE END OF YOUR SECOND
7-DAY WEIGHED FOOD SURVEY

The data is required to evaluate the effort and changes in lifestyle involved in trying to modify your eating habits.

Please answer the following questions by placing a tick or answer in the relevant brackets, or commenting as appropriate.

A 1 Did you enjoy your food this week:

As much as usual?   ( )

More than usual?   ( )
Less than usual?   ( )

2a Could the last seven days diet (i.e., during the weighed food survey) become a permanent way of life? (As long as you didn't have to weigh everything?)

Yes   ( )
No   ( )
Uncertain   ( )

2b Please comment _____

_____

_____

B WHEN MODIFYING YOUR EATING HABITS DURING THIS SECOND SURVEY WEEK:-

1 Did other members of your household eat meals similar to yours?

Yes   ( )
No   ( )
Uncertain   ( )
N/A   ( )

Please comment _____

_____

2a Did you deliberately use different or adapted recipes or ingredients from usual (consider your own recipes as well as published ones)?

Yes   ( )
No   ( )

2b Did you alter your cooking *methods*?

Yes   ( )
No   ( )
Uncertain   ( )

3a Did you deliberately eat food bought from shops other than your regular ones?

Yes   ( )
No   ( )
Uncertain   ( )

3b Where did you do the shopping for the food you *ate* during the past seven days?
Please indicate the shop used most frequently as 1, the next as 2, etc., for all shops used.

SCORE

Usual supermarket ( )
Different supermarket ( )
Small general grocers ( )
Traditional shops e.g. butcher, baker, grocer ( )
Market ( )
Health Food Shop ( )
Ethnic shop i.e. Indian/Chinese ( )
Wholefood grocers ( )
Others, please specify _____

3c Compared to usual was shopping for the foods you *ate* this week:

More convenient ( )
More difficult ( )
No different ( )

4 Did you find that the availability of suitable pre-prepared foods affected your efforts to eat a healthy diet?

Adversely ( )
Advantageously ( )
Uncertain ( )
Not at all ( )

5 How long each day did you spend in preparing the food you ate and clearing up (excluding the time spent recording data for this survey)? Please give your best estimate ..... hrs/mins

6a Are there any factors that limited the enjoyment of the food you ate? e.g. time, availability of foods, cost, knowledge about food, etc?

Yes ( )
No ( )
Uncertain ( )

6b Please comment _____

_____

7 Do you think the amount you spent on food was, compared with usual:

Increased? ( )
Decreased? ( )
About the same? ( )

8a Did the amount and/or type of your social activities change?

Yes ( )
No ( )

8b If 'yes' please specify nature of change _____

_____

9 Did the number of meals you ate in the office/works canteen:

Increase?	( )
Decrease?	( )
Remain about the same?	( )
Uncertain?	( )

10 Did the number of meals you ate in restaurants or out socially:

Increase?	( )
Decrease?	( )
Remain about the same?	( )
Uncertain?	( )

11 Weight at the end of the week
..... st ..... lbs   OR ..... kgs

_____

C This section is optional and aimed at covering any pertinent points not covered by sections A & B.
  1 Please contribute your experience and comments on modifying your eating habits to achieve any of the following guidelines:-
    FIBRE _____

    _____

    _____

    _____

    FAT _____

    _____

    _____

    _____

    SUGAR _____

    _____

    _____

    ALCOHOL _____

    _____

    _____

    _____

SALT _____

_____

_____

_____

2 Any other comments? _____

_____

_____

_____

Please do not feel restricted by the spaces provided. Feel free to attach extra notes if you wish.

THANK YOU FOR YOUR HELP

SAMPLE OF A SECOND NUTRITION ASSESSMENT (FOR A MALE PARTICIPANT)

Dear Participant,   27/10/84

Thank you for the second record of your food intake. We have attempted to compare your data with a focus on the targets set by NACNE using the same guidelines as before. Again, we have not included your Plurivite in the analysis.

Section 1. YOUR PERSONAL DATA. The data you reported is shown below:

Age	31 years
Height	173cms
Weight	62.0Kg
Frame size	Medium

According to the Metropolitan Life Insurance Company (1983), your weight is 4.5 per cent below the lower limit desirable (65.5 – 71.0kg) for your height and frame size.

Section 2. SUMMARY OF PARTICIPATION

		First record	Second record	NACNE guideline
Fibre	g	22.6	41.4	=>30.0
Sodium	mg	2929.4	3194.7	<3600
Sugar	% Kcals.	15.0	7.1	<10
Saturated fat	% Kcals.	15.9	7.3	<10
Total fat	% Kcals.	37.1	27.1	<30
Alcohol	% Kcals.	1.0	2.0	<8

YOUR ACHIEVEMENT OF THE NACNE GUIDELINES

Thank you for all that hard work! We congratulate you on your achievements. Your second analysis indicates that you have made a considerable effort to attain the NACNE dietary guidelines for this assessment. The interesting point now is can you keep them up!

Do please bear in mind that while NACNE has provided us with useful guidelines, we by no means know all the answers to diet in relation to health. We should also remember that the NACNE recommendations are based on averages for the whole population.

Section 3. YOUR DIETARY/NUTRIENT BREAKDOWN
The nutrients provided by the food and beverage items you reported are shown below and compared with the recommended daily intake for a group of people your sex, age and activity level:

Nutrient	Unit	First Daily Intake	Second Daily Intake	Recommended Daily Requirements	References
Energy	Calorie	2306.7	1960.9	2510.0	1
Protein	g	78.5	97.0	63.0	1
Fat (Total)	g	95.0	59.0	<30% Kcal.	2,3
Carbohydrate (Total)	g	297.0	267.3	###	
Sugars (Total)	g	166.8	111.9	###	
Fibre	g	22.6	41.4	30.0	2
Potassium	mg	3255.2	4621.8	###	
Calcium	mg	955.4	1222.3	500.0	1
Iron	mg	13.0	16.1	10.0	1
Zinc	mg	10.7	14.1	15.0	4

Nutrient	Unit	First Daily Intake	Second Daily Intake	Recommended Daily Requirements	References
Sodium	mg	2929.4	3194.7	<3600	2,3
Vitamin A (RE)	mcg	981.9	889.6	750.0	1
Carotene	mcg	2366.0	2041.3	###	
Vitamin D	mcg	5.4	6.0	Sunlight!	1
Vitamin E	mg	6.0	7.2	15.0	4
Vitamin B12	mcg	3.9	4.8	3.0	4
Riboflavin	mg	2.2	2.9	1.6	1
Niacin (NE)	mg	38.2	47.4	18.0	1
Vitamin C	mg	91.7	161.5	30.0	1
Vitamin B6	mg	1.4	2.4	2.0	4
Folic acid	mcg	158.8	324.3	300.0	1
Cholesterol	mg	373.6	174.2	<300	3,5
Saturated fat	% of Kcals.	15.9	7.3	<10	2,3,5
Essential PUFAs	% of Kcals.	5.4	9.2	>3	5
P/S Ratio		.3	1.3	1.0	2,5
% Kcalories from protein		13.6	19.8		
% Kcalories from fat		37.1	27.1	<30	2,3
% Kcalories from carbohydrate		48.3	51.1		
% Kcalories from added sugars		15.0	7.1	<10	2
% Kcalories from alcohol		1.0	2.0	<8	based on 2,3,6

[### no recommended figure has been set.]

References

1. DHSS Report on Health and Social Subjects No. 15. 1979. Recommended Daily Amounts of Food Energy and Nutrients for Groups of People in the United Kingdom. HMSO.
2. Health Education Council 1983. Proposals for Nutritional Guidelines for Health Education in Britain. A discussion paper.
3. WHO 1982. 'Prevention of Coronary heart disease' Technical report series 678. WHO, Geneva.
4. National Research Council, National Academy of Sciences: Recommended Daily Dietary Allowances. Revised 1974.
5. FAO/WHO 1978 'Dietary fats and oils in human nutrition' Nutrition report no.3 FAO, Rome.
6. DHSS Report on Health and Social Subjects, no.28. 1984. 'Diet and cardiovascular disease' HMSO, London.

Section 4. ASSESSMENT OF YOUR DIETARY INTAKE

This second assessment provides you with information on the extent to which you have achieved the NACNE targets and also on most of the nutrients thought to be important to health. The main purpose of this second analysis is to consider how far you have met the NACNE long term guidelines:-

SODIUM: Congratulations, your sodium intake has remained below the long term NACNE recommended upper level of 3600 mg/day. Remember however, that the analysis does not take into account salt added in cooking and/or at table. As you state you do not add salt your intake should remain within the guideline set by NACNE.

Interestingly, in a recent study by Claudia Sanchez-Castillo and Phillip James on 116 people, only 11.6 per cent of their salt intake came from added salt (6.5 per cent from table salt and 5.1 per cent from salt added in cooking), while 88.4 per cent was provided from food and drink i.e. non-discretionary sources (Nut. Soc. April 1984). So, whilst it is prudent to avoid adding extra salt to food at table and in cooking perhaps more importantly, fresh food should be eaten where possible, thus avoiding too many processed foods. It also highlights the limited value of expensive salt substitutes if processed foods are not avoided.

FIBRE: Congratulations! Your fibre intake is now above the recommended level of 30g/day. As a matter of interest, check to see if your vitamin and mineral intakes have also improved.

SUCROSE: Well done! You have managed to reduce your intake of sucrose and refined sugars to within the guidelines set by NACNE.

ALCOHOL: The NACNE recommendations on alcohol intakes refer to 20g per day (4 per cent of the dietary energy) per head of the population which was the average consumption in the 1960's; but this is a mean value for all which includes infants, children and those who do not drink. We suggested in the first assessment that a realistic interpretation of this might be that it would be wise to keep alcohol consumption to below 8 per cent of your energy. Your intake therefore, has remained at a satisfactory level. We are pleased that the efforts of attaining the guidelines has not driven you to drink . . . excessively, at least!

FAT: Congratulations, you have achieved the NACNE long term target. This is a considerable achievement on your part, well done. Now, can you keep it up!

SATURATED FAT: Well done, you have managed to reduce your saturated fat intake to a satisfactory level. This seems to be a particularly difficult target to meet so you have done very well. In reducing your saturated fat your P/S ratio has also improved considerably.

Section 5. PREVENTION OF CARDIOVASCULAR DISEASE

In the response to your first record we mentioned the need for attention to the prevention of heart disease which is the single most important cause of death in this country. Atherosclerosis and thrombosis are the underlying features and both are influenced by long term nutritional and lifestyle considerations. Their influence is not, however, restricted to the heart but can impair the function of other vascular systems such as the kidneys, brain and reproductive system. Consequently, the nutritional and lifestyle principles behind the prevention of heart disease are important to general health and the quality of life: in different ways, they are of equal significance to men and women.

The following table considers the lifestyle choices that you have made and your family history that should be taken into account when planning your personal health care programme.

1. DIET		We acknowledge the changes you have made in attempting to achieve the dietary goals.
2. SMOKING	NO:	A health bonus! Your risk of dying from a heart attack is ten times less than that of a heavy smoker.
3. FAMILY HISTORY OF CHD	YES:	No-one can choose their genetic make-up but it can be taken as an early warning light and preventative steps are particularly important in your case.
4. OVERWEIGHT	NO:	A health bonus!
5. EXERCISE	NO:	In a study carried out in America, the risk of death from ischaemic heart disease was found to be almost three times greater in inactive men than in those who participated in some form of regular exercise. Exercise also improves general physical well-being. It is important to take

part in some form of regular
exercise which you enjoy and
which increases your pulse rate.

6. STRESS   NO: A health bonus! While stress may
not cause the disease to the
arteries and blood which leads to
heart attacks, it is believed to be
important in the timing of an
attack.

7. HYPERTENSION   NO: A health bonus! Keep it that way.

Section 6. AFTER NACNE

It is of interest that since the beginning of this programme, the DHSS
has published the report of its Committee on Medical Aspects of Food
Policy (COMA). The recommendations made in this report reinforce
those of NACNE on the need to reduce fats, particularly saturated
fats, although they are made with less vigour.

Committees of National and International status have made recommendations that are similar to those of NACNE and COMA. Positive
health promotion, as well as prevention of heart disease is clearly
multifactorial, both in the dietary sense as well as in lifestyle. Some fat
in the diet is required to provide the essential polyunsaturated fatty
acids needed for cell regulation and platelet function, and as a vehicle
for fat soluble vitamins. Excess sugar is rapidly absorbed, stimulates
insulin secretion and is converted to fat, mainly of a saturated nature.
The interaction between sugars and fats have wide ranging metabolic
effects which are of particular relevance to the regulation of hormone
secretion. There is now evidence on the role of dietary fibre in the
function of the large bowel and in cholesterol excretion.

The issue of nutrition influencing long term biology will become of
greater significance when the debate on nutrition and cancer enters a
more public arena. In 1982 the National Academy of Sciences of the
USA reviewed the question of nutrition and cancer. The conclusion
was drawn that a substantial part of cancer, particularly breast and
colon cancer was related to food; again, diets high in fats and purified
carbohydrates appeared to be strongly correlated. This conclusion
was drawn by Sir Richard Doll in 1968 but most of the attention to
his writings was devoted to the single issue of smoking and lung
cancer. The question of nutrition and cancer prevention is now being
seriously considered by the National Cancer Institute of the USA and
will almost inevitably have an influence on thinking on this side of the
Atlantic.

It is a general principle from experimental nutrition, that nutritional deficits or imbalances have their most profound effects during periods of growth. This principle applies just as much to early human growth and development. There is now evidence which indicates that development during early childhood and even fetal growth can be critical in determining health in later life. Two of the major risk factors – raised blood lipids and the increase in blood pressure – are already detectable by seven years of age in children from populations at high risk of heart disease.

It is likely that nutrition will need to play an increasingly important role as an active force in promoting good health. Having noticed how many of the participants have frequently adopted a positive approach in attempting to achieve the NACNE guidelines, we hope that Dietitians and Nutritionists will be able to encourage this practice of focusing on foods which are beneficial rather than the negative attitude of denial. The idea of 'what should not be eaten' is often linked with non-adherence; on the other hand, an emphasis on the diversity of foods which are useful, must add to the social pleasures of eating and the enjoyment of life.

We wish to thank you for contributing to this research project, which we hope has been of use to you personally and professionally. We have found the dietary records and questionnaires to be most interesting. They have generated a substantial volume of data which will illustrate the issues involved in achieving the dietary goals.

In the meantime, we would very much appreciate any comments or suggestions you may have, which would help to improve the use of this programme. Comments would be welcomed on the style and content of the programme including ways of suggesting dietary modifications. We would be especially interested to hear of techniques that you may have used to help meet at least some of the NACNE guidelines.

References

1. Doll, R., Muir, C. & Waterhouse J. 1966. Cancer Incidence in Five Continents. Springer-Verlag, New York.
2. Committee on Diet, Nutrition and Cancer. 1982. Assembly of Life Sciences, National Research Council. National Academy Press, Washington, D.C.

We hope you have enjoyed participating in this assessment of your nutritional status and we wish you the best of health. We look forward to sharing the results with you in the near future.

This analysis is provided by the Flora Project for Heart Disease Prevention, using data supplied by the Department of Biochemistry and Nutrition at The Nuffield Laboratories of Comparative Medicine, McCance & Widdowson's 'The Composition of Foods' and the American Department of Agriculture.

Some Useful Sources of Information

A Discussion Paper on Proposals for Nutritional Guidelines for Health Education in Britain, prepared for the National Advisory Committee on Nutrition Education (NACNE) by an ad hoc working party under the Chairmanship of Professor W. P. T. James. London, Health Education Council, 1983

Diet and Cardiovascular Disease. Department of Health & Social Security, Committee on Medical Aspects of Food Policy: Report on Health & Social Subjects No. 28, London, HMSO, 1984

Recommended Daily Amount of Food Energy and Nutrients for Groups of People in the United Kingdom. Department of Health & Social Security, Report on Health & Social Subjects No. 15, London, HMSO, 1979

The Food Scandal. Caroline Walker and Geoffrey Cannon, London, Century Publishing, 1984

McCance and Widdowson's The Composition of Foods. ed. Paul A. A. & Southgate D. A. T. ed. 4th Edition, London, HMSO, 1978

Present Day Practice in Infant Feeding. DHSS Report No. 20, 1980

Artificial Feeds for the Young Infant. DHSS Report No. 18, 1980

Towards a Sugar Health Policy. Sanderson M., MSc Thesis, Cranfield Institute of Technology, 1984

Prevention of Coronary Heart Disease. WHO Expert Committee, Technical Report Series, London, HMSO, 1982

Index